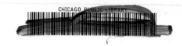

Health Care of Homeless People

Philip W. Brickner, M.D., is a graduate of Columbia University College of Physicians and Surgeons. He is an Internist and has been Director of the Department of Community Medicine at Saint Vincent's Hospital and Medical Center of New York since 1974. The Department of Community Medicine has among its goals the seeking out and assisting of medically unreached people in New York City, including the homeless, the frail, the homebound aged, and immigrant children. Dr. Brickner is the author of numerous articles on these subjects in the professional literature.

Linda Keen Scharer, M.U.P., received her master's degree in urban planning from New York University. She is presently Assistant Director of the Department of Community Medicine at St. Vincent's Hospital and Medical Center of New York. In addition to her work with the homeless, Ms. Scharer has written extensively on home health care issues and serves on the editorial board of the PRIDE Institute *Journal of Long-Term Home Health Care*.

Barbara Conanan, R.N., M.S., is Director of the SRO/Homeless Program within the Department of Community Medicine at Saint Vincent's Hospital and Medical Center of New York. She has served in this capacity since January 1983. In addition, Ms. Conanan gives direct patient care as a Community Health Nurse. Prior to her employment at St. Vincent's, she worked at the Manhattan Bowery Corporation as supervisor in an outpatient clinic that provided services to chronic alcoholics.

Alexander Elvy, M.S.W., is a Certified Social Worker who graduated from the Columbia University School of Social Work in 1970. Since then, Mr. Elvy has held numerous positions as a program developer and community organizer. He has worked extensively with local community organizations throughout New York City, and has served as a Board member of the New York City Coalition for the Homeless since its founding in 1980. Presently, Mr. Elvy holds the staff position of Social Worker/Community Organizer in the Department of Community Medicine at St. Vincent's Hospital and Medical Center of New York.

Marianne Savarese, R.N., B.S.N., is a graduate of St. Vincent's Hospital School of Nursing and received a bachelor of science degree in nursing from Adelphi University. For the past five years she has been a Community Health Nurse member of an interdisciplinary team at the Department of Community Medicine, St. Vincent's Hospital, providing health care to homeless women at a New York City shelter.

Health Care of Homeless People

Philip W. Brickner, M.D.
Linda Keen Scharer, M.U.P.
Barbara Conanan, R.N., M.S.
Alexander Elvy, M.S.W.
Marianne Savarese, R.N., B.S.N.

Editors

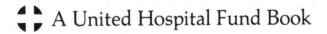 A United Hospital Fund Book

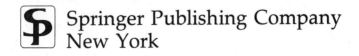 Springer Publishing Company
New York

Springer Publishing Company, Inc.
536 Broadway
New York, New York 10012

85 86 87 88 89 / 10 9 8 7 6 5 4 3 2

Library of Congress Cataloging in Publication Data

Main entry under title:

Health care of homeless people.
  Includes bibliographies and index.
  1. Homelessness—Hygienic aspects—United States—Addresses, essays, lectures.
2. Poor—Medical care—United States—Addresses, essays, lectures.   3. Mentally
ill—Care and treatment—United States—Addresses, essays, lectures.   I. Brickner,
Philip W.
RA770.H43   1985   362.1'0425   84-23625
ISBN 0-8261-4990-1

Printed in the United States of America

Contents _____

Part III   MENTAL HEALTH AND ILLNESS

Part IV   ORGANIZATION OF HEALTH CARE SERVICES

Part V VIABLE MODELS

Foreword

Nothing reveals the paradoxes of contemporary health care in the United States better than the medical problems of the homeless. Our modern medical centers are equipped with esoteric technologies that enable the staff to perform miraculous cures. We can transplant kidneys and livers, implant prosthetic hips, and cure an increasing fraction of cancers. Yet literally within shouting distance of these centers, the socially and economically displaced are afflicted with conditions no longer commonly perceived as major problems in our country. While tuberculosis, skin ulceration, and malnutrition are routinely preventable or easily treated in the general population, they remain relatively serious issues among the homeless. The most difficult problems are not posed by science, but by the political, organizational, and economic mechanisms that separate the technological capacity to treat or cure and those who desperately need treatment and curing.

Since 1879, the United Hospital Fund of New York has sought to support and ensure comprehensive, high-quality health care delivery. As a research, planning, and educational institution, the Fund has encouraged the creation or improvement of existing mechanisms that effectively deliver health care to sick people. As an initiator and leader in health care policy, the Fund has sought to identify and define pressing issues susceptible to effective intervention and to assemble those best able to address them. As a federated philanthropy, the Fund has directed its resources to those institutions that possess the technical capacity to provide care but are fiscally constrained from caring for those unable to pay.

Participating in the production of this volume is a logical extension of that commitment. We hope it will be an important contribution to the essential process of improving health care for extremely needy people.

Bruce C. Vladeck, Ph.D.
President
The United Hospital Fund
of New York
New York, New York

Preface

The information available about the health problems of homeless people is rudimentary. The attention of those concerned with the homeless has, quite properly, been focused upon housing and food. Yet matters of health and illness are of major importance, both to the individuals directly at risk and to the general public.

This book is an attempt to put forward fundamental data on the subject. It is intended to serve as a guide for physicians, nurses, social workers, shelter staff members, and program managers who work with the homeless; to suggest approaches for the development and conduct of health-related programs in shelters and other places where homeless people congregate; and to be a resource for hospital administrators, voluntary agencies, and policy makers in government who have an obligation to help meet the health care needs of the homeless.

The authors of this book have worked with the homeless in cities across the country. They are professionals in relevant disciplines, creators of programs, innovators in government. Their direct experience in planning for and giving care is chronicled here, directly on the record, for the use of others.

The first section defines the homeless and introduces the subject of health care for these people, gives historical background and dimension to the issue, and places appropriate focus on the problem of chronicity in regard to their health problems.

The second section is concerned with medical disorders. The illnesses of homeless people are common problems aggravated by the style of life they are forced to lead. Esoteric diseases are not the issue here. We are working instead with infections, infestations, trauma, the consequences of poor nutrition, peripheral vascular disease, alcoholism, and tuberculosis.

The third section comprises information on mental health and mental illness in homeless people. The incidence of psychiatric disease is high in this group, requires serious attention, and places major demands on health care personnel.

The fourth section covers the organization of health care programs, understanding how to help the homeless obtain access to medical coverage and services, and developing networks among local agencies, hospitals, and government.

The final section focuses on viable program models. These examples show how people with energy and a desire to help can generate effective results. Partnerships and coalitions can, in fact, overcome divisiveness, disputes over authority, and lack of funds to achieve common goals if motivation is sufficiently strong.

Serious problems exist in the field of health care for the homeless. The few programs now functioning are hardly sufficient to meet the need. This book may provide the stimulus necessary to develop more programs. Our country and its people are now suffering the onerous consequences of earlier social policy decisions. Among these are real estate practices in major urban areas that have allowed low-cost housing to shrivel or disappear; economic planning that has led to structural unemployment, especially among young minority-group people; and the enforced deinstitutionalization from state hospitals of the chronically mentally ill. Thousands of these individuals are now helpless in the streets of our cities.

Total solutions to these complex problems are not evident today. We have, instead, an opportunity to work together in tangible ways, with local resources, to help people in need. The homeless are human beings who deserve help. We can offer assistance, and should do so.

Philip W. Brickner
Linda Keen Scharer
Barbara Conanan
Alexander Elvy
Marianne Savarese

Acknowledgments

The development of this work was nurtured by the United Hospital Fund of New York. The Fund sponsored a national conference on Health Issues in the Care of the Homeless in October 1983, from which the text's concept emerged. The Fund is responsible for significant financial support of this book as well. The Pew Memorial Trust has also given noteworthy backing. The editors are deeply grateful to the United Hospital Fund and to the Pew Memorial Trust for their help in this regard.

We wish to thank the authors who participated in the creation of this volume. These people, leaders in the field of health care for the homeless, put forth great effort, under considerable pressure of time, to prepare their work for this purpose.

We owe special thanks to Michelle Salcedo for editing; to Daniel Beaudoin for work on the bibliographies; to Patricia Ambrosino for word processing; and to Robert Markel of Markel Enterprises for agenting. Bruce Vladeck, Dina Keller, and Sally Rogers of the United Hospital Fund of New York, Rebecca Rimel of the Pew Memorial Trust, and Barbara Watkins and Elizabeth Corra of Springer Publishing have been particularly helpful in bringing this complex project to fruition.

Our own institution, St. Vincent's Hospital and Medical Center of New York, has been a major force in developing health care programs for the homeless. Since 1969 people from St. Vincent's have been working in Manhattan's shelters and single-room-occupancy hotels. These efforts are a logical function of our hospital, which was founded in 1849 by the Sisters of Charity of St. Vincent de Paul to care for the sick poor. We wish to acknowledge the magnificent service given to the homeless through these programs, both at shelter sites and within the hospital, by many staff members; and it gives us particular pleasure to thank individuals within the administration and professional staff of our hospital who have encouraged these efforts: the late Sister Anthony Marie FitzMaurice, Sister Evelyn Schneider, Sister Margaret Sweeney, Sister Marian Catherine Muldoon, Albert Samis, Gary Horan, Tom Mc-Gourty, John Fales, Jack Koretsky, Ed Cagan, Steve Wobido, Debra Oryzysyn, Paulette Ortiz, Ray Rodriquez, John Ferguson, Joe Corcoran, Roger Weaving, Martin Spector, Jeff Davis, Maryann Maisonet, Joe English, James Mazzara, Joe Hoffman, Ted Druhot, Jeff Naiditch, Sister Margaret Murphy, Anthony Lechich, Arthur Kaufman, Darcy Guhl, Agnes Frank, Rhona Kelley, Mary Hart, Laura Starita, and James Janeski.

Contributors

Eve Bargmann, M.D.
Zacchaeus Clinic
Washington, D.C.

Gay Lynn Bond, M.S.W.
Director of Social Services
Charity Hospital
New Orleans, La.

Laura Cavicci, R.N.
Head Nurse
Boston Shelter for the Homeless
Boston, Mass.

Stephanie Cowles, M.S.W.
Director, West Side Social Setting
Alcoholism Treatment Program
Manhattan Bowery Corporation
New York, N.Y.

Sister Julie Crane, R.N., F.N.P.
Sisters of Providence Health Care
  for the Homeless
Springfield, Mass.

Stephen Crystal, Ph.D.
Director, Bureau of Management
  Systems, Planning, Research, and
  Evaluation
Family and Adult Services
Human Resources Administration
New York, N.Y.

Patricia Doherty, R.N.
Head Nurse, Keener Building
SRO/Homeless Program
Department of Community
  Medicine
St. Vincent's Hospital and
  Medical Center of New York
New York, N.Y.

Dearborn Edwards, M.D.
Fellow in Immunology
University of Colorado School of
  Medicine
Denver, Colo.
(Formerly Physician, Department
  of Community Medicine, St.
  Vincent's Hospital and Medical
  Center of New York,
  New York, N.Y.)

Brian Fallon, M.Ed.
4th-Year Medical Student
Columbia University College of
  Physicians and Surgeons
New York, N.Y.

Thomas Filardo, M.D.
Assistant Professor in Family
  Practice
University of Illinois College of
  Medicine at Urbana/Champaign
Urbana, Ill.

Kevin Flynn, Ph.D.
Los Angeles County Department of
  Mental Health
Civic Center Project
Los Angeles, Calif.

Edward I. Geffner, J.D.
Executive Director, Manhattan
  Bowery Corporation
New York, N.Y.

Roslynn Glicksman, M.D.
Peace Corps
(Formerly Resident Physician,
  Department of Community
  Medicine, St. Vincent's Hospital
  and Medical Center of New York,
  New York, N.Y.)

Lewis Goldfrank, M.D.
Director
Emergency Services
Bellevue and University Hospitals
New York, N.Y.

Richard W. Green, M.D.
Clinical Associate Professor in
    Dermatology
New York University Medical Center
New York, N.Y.

Ronnie S. Halper, M.S.W., M.P.H.
Program Analyst
New York City Department of
    Mental Health, Mental Retarda-
    tion and Alcoholism Services
New York, N.Y.

Barbara Henley, M.S.W.
Director, Department of Social
    Work
Ben Taub Hospital
Houston, Tex.

Marybeth Hopkins, M.S.W.
Senior Program Analyst
New York City Department of
    Mental Health, Mental Retarda-
    tion and Alcoholism Services
New York, N.Y.

Michael Iseman, M.D.
Associate Professor of Medicine
Division of Pulmonary Sciences
University of Colorado School of
    Medicine
Denver, Colo.

Sara L. Kellermann, M.D.
Commissioner
New York City Department of
    Mental Health
Mental Retardation and Alcoholism
    Services
New York, N.Y.

F. Russell Kellogg, M.D.
Attending Physician
Department of Community
    Medicine
St. Vincent's Hospital and
    Medical Center of New York
New York, N.Y.

John T. Kelly, M.D., Ph.D.
Medical Director
Medically Indigent Adult Program
Department of Public Health
San Francisco, Calif.

Elizabeth Kiernan, R.N.
Director of Nursing Services
Manhattan Bowery Corporatioᵢ
New York, N.Y.

Litrelle T. Levy, M.S.W.
Assistant Director
Department of Social Work
Ben Taub Hospital
Houston, Tex.

Monica Mang, B.S.
Human Service Worker
Social Service Psychiatry Unit
Charity Hospital
New Orleans, La.

John McAdam, M.D.
Attending Physician
SRO/Homeless Program
Department of Community
    Medicine
St. Vincent's Hospital and
    Medical Center of New York
New York, N.Y.

Kevin McBride, M.D.
Fellow in Peripheral Vascular
    Surgery
Boston University
Boston, Mass.

Barbara N. McInnes, R.N.
Pine Street Inn
Boston, Mass.

Robert Morgan, M.D.
Attending Physician
Department of Medicine
St. Vincent's Hospital and
 Medical Center of New York
New York, N.Y.

Robert J. Mulcare, M.D.
Attending Surgeon
St. Luke's–Roosevelt Hospital
 Center
Chief, Vascular Service
Roosevelt Division
New York, N.Y.

Gail B. Nayowith, M.S.W.
Senior Rehabilitation Specialist
New York City Department of
 Mental Health, Mental Retarda-
 tion and Alcoholism Services
New York, N.Y.

John Noble, M.D.
Professor of Medicine
Boston University School of
 Medicine
Chief, Section of General Internal
 Medicine
Boston City Hospital
Boston, Mass.

Mary Jean O'Brien, R.N., M.Ed.
Supervisor of Nursing
Department of Community
 Medicine
St. Vincent's Hospital and
 Medical Center of New York
New York, N.Y.

Olga Piantieri, R.N.
SRO/Homeless Program
Department of Community
 Medicine
St. Vincent's Hospital and
 Medical Center of New York
New York, N.Y.

Bart Price, B.B.A., C.P.A.
Chief Financial Officer
Yale–New Haven Hospital
New Haven, Conn.

Eileen Reilly, R.N.
Clinic Administrator
Pine Street Inn
Boston, Mass.

Paul E. Robinson
Deputy Commissioner for
 Addiction Services
Boston, Mass.

Thomas Scott
Shelter Director
Boston Shelter for the Homeless
Boston, Mass.

William J. Vicic, M.D.
Attending Physician
SRO/Homeless Program
Department of Community
 Medicine
St. Vincent's Hospital and
 Medical Center of New York
New York, N.Y.

Karen Wilkinson, M.P.A.
Administrative Resident
Charity Hospital
New Orleans, La.

Myron Winick, M.D.
R.R. Williams Professor of
  Nutrition and Pediatrics
Director, Institute of Human
  Nutrition
Columbia University College of
  Physicians and Surgeons
New York, N.Y.

Philip Yanowitch, M.A.
2nd-Year Medical Student
Downstate Medical Center School
  of Medicine
Brooklyn, N.Y.

PART I

INTRODUCTION

1

Health Issues in the Care of the Homeless

Philip W. Brickner

> For every hour and every moment thousands of men leave life on this earth, and their souls appear before God. And how many of them depart in solitude, unknown, sad, dejected, that no one mourns for them or even knows whether they have lived or not.[1]

The medical disorders of the homeless are all the ills to which flesh is heir, magnified by disordered living conditions, exposure to extremes of heat and cold, lack of protection from rain and snow, bizarre sleeping accommodations, and overcrowding in shelters. These factors are exacerbated by stress, psychiatric disorders, and sociopathic behavior patterns.

A caveat: shelter and food are the prime needs of homeless people; health matters, important as they are, generally follow next.

Why are we concerned about the health of homeless people? A straightforward desire to help others in trouble is part of the answer; a wish to make our society as humane as we can. Public health issues arise as well; for example, the persistence of pulmonary tuberculosis in this group means a pool of infection that can spread outward.[2-4]

The information base about health problems of the homeless is rudimentary. During our attempts to learn about earlier work in the field, we have discovered a virtual library of sociological texts[5,6] based

3

upon the romance of skid row. Studies of derelicts have produced many a Ph.D. thesis. In all this work, however, there is rarely a comment about health or disease. The same vacuum exists in the 957 pages of the 1982 *Congressional Hearing on Homelessness in America.*[7]

DEFINING THE HOMELESS

The number of homeless people in our country is not known.[8,9] Without doubt, from the time our species has existed, individuals handicapped by physical or emotional disorders, addiction, societal prejudice and/or aberrant behavior have tended to slide to the bottom of the social scale. Since cities have existed, such people have congregated in the least expensive, most deteriorated areas, where conduct and appearance that would not be tolerated elsewhere are accepted. These people are unlikely to be recorded in any census. They are not domiciled, tend to avoid answering questions, and are often afraid, suspicious, or angry.

The present surge of interest in the homeless is laudable by any measure, but the size of the problem may not in fact be news. In New York City, recent estimates are that the homeless may number as many as 36,000.[10-12] This figure, although of uncertain validity,[13] compares interestingly with the 1964 survey data prepared by George Nash of Columbia University:[5] Manhattan had at least 30,000 homeless men not on the Bowery; a Bowery count added 7,611 more.

The concern about homeless persons is worldwide, as studies from Sweden,[14] Canada,[15] and England[16] indicate. A case in point is the Soviet Union, where "winos" are commonplace—dotting the pavements, staggering through crowds, accosting passersby.[17]

Random distribution of any large population will leave a proportion at the lowest end. Is the figure in the United States 1 percent? If so, there are about 2.4 million homeless. Is it 0.5 percent? Then the homeless number about 1.2 million. Federal government estimates that there are about a quarter of a million homeless persons in the country[18] are probably an understatement.

Our definition of the homeless in this discussion includes:

- skid row people;
- patients discharged from mental hospitals;
- the new homeless, purportedly without shelter because they are economic casualties;
- homeless youth;
- homeless women.

We must add those who are living isolated lives in rooming houses and single-room-occupancy (SRO) hotels. In those inner city areas where the phenomenon of gentrification is taking place, SRO residents are at risk of homelessness. Furthermore, the similarities of personal conduct and illness between truly homeless individuals and those in marginal housing are striking.[19]

SKID ROW

Skid row has come to mean the sections of a city where the down-and-out cluster.[20] The term derives from Skid Road in Seattle, where logging teams pulled their loads to a mill.[21] "This street became the locus for cheap bars, cheap entertainment and cheap lodgings."[12] *Skid row*, or *skid road*, as a term, has assumed highly attractive metaphorical qualities. It stands for a downhill course of life that is out of control.

Bogue estimated in 1963[22] that at least fifty cities in America had identifiable skid rows. This figure is probably acceptable today,[23,24] although skid row itself has changed over the years. As Hopper and Baxter point out:

> . . . the new skid row has as its most obvious feature the distinction that it is no longer confined to well-demarcated "tenderloin" areas of large cities. In most places, the homeless have ceased to observe the old strict geographical bounds. In New York City, the streets and subways, doorways and alleyways, public parks and transportation depots are home for thousands of our citizens each night.[10]

Rough estimates suggest that about one-fifth of homeless people are skid row persons,[5] largely men who have sunk to the bottom of the social scale: chronic alcoholics, derelicts, chronic psychotics. Generalizations of this sort are, of course, highly simplistic and suspect; demographics shift, neighborhoods change,[6] definitions are inaccurate, and overlapping occurs.

PATIENTS DISCHARGED FROM
MENTAL HOSPITALS

Schizophrenia and other major psychiatric disorders are significantly overrepresented among the homeless.[15,25-30] Where do these people come from?

By the mid-twentieth century, mental hospitals had become recognized as institutions inherently custodial in nature. Attempts to cure patients of psychiatric disease were ineffective, and costs of care were high. These hospitals, and the government policies that sustained them, were perceived increasingly as mechanisms for social control without due process. A consensus grew in favor of a new, nonhospital mode of treatment that would require a spirit of humaneness, public favor, and financial feasibility. The harsh, custodial spirit was to be changed into one of kindness and warmth.[31]

In about 1955,[30] the community psychiatry movement, in association with public advocates and civil libertarians, initiated a process that led to the discharge into the community of patients from state mental hospitals. State governments, perceiving the potential for cost decreases, were willing partners in this effort. The numbers of state psychiatric hospital patients in the United States, at a peak of 558,992 in 1955,[32] had fallen to 248,518 by 1973,[33] had reached a figure of about 146,000 in 1979,[34] and is thought to be at a level of 132,000 in 1984.[35] Community care was presumed preferable to incarceration. Through this process the accepted public policy goals[31] for the mentally ill were to be retained:

- protection of dependent people as a humanitarian act;
- social control of deviant individuals;
- seeking cure of disease at an acceptable dollar cost.

The design for services, as alternatives to state hospitals, was to include care in community mental health centers, outpatient departments, family care homes, halfway houses, psychiatric beds in community hospitals for crises, after-care provided by psychiatric social workers and community-oriented psychiatrists, and sheltered workshops.

The discovery of new medications was a potent element in this design. Psychotropic drugs such as chlorpromazine (Thorazine) were felt to offer the ideal of therapy: humane treatment instead of custody, social control, and low cost. These drugs ''promoted psychiatrists to physicians in the eyes of some of their colleagues, and the insane to the status of patients in the eyes of many members of the public.''[36]

It is evident to any observer of the passing scene that this attractive theoretical plan has failed to a significant degree. Numerous, although uncounted, psychotic people are suffering on the streets and in shelters without adequate mental health services. A careful analysis in a major New York City shelter for the homeless[29] revealed that one-third of the residents present for two months or more had a prior history of state hospitalization. Others were psychiatrically ill, but without a record. The process of state hospital discharge, which started more than twenty years ago, continues. (See Table 1.1.)

Restrictive admission policies deny many chronic psychotic patients the opportunity to return to state institutions on those unfortunate occasions when placement appears to be the best option. The road back to the mental hospital is nearly closed.[31]

Why has the community psychiatry movement failed these people? Segal and Aviram, in an admirable summary,[31] point out that a major reason is community opposition to placement. Fear of the mentally ill, sense of threat about behavior and conduct, and anxiety about loss of local property values are present. Exclusionary laws to inhibit sheltered community housing have been created. Informal mechanisms are developed for stalling, including "impossible" fire permit regulations. As a result, former mental patients, unwelcome and impoverished, drift into skid row and ghetto areas, the streets and shelters.

States have issued regulations to deal with the consequences of deinstitutionalization. However, funds have not been made available to fulfill these regulations, and motivation may be lacking as well. The results are present for all to see.

Irony abounds. Manhattan State Hospital on Ward's Island in New York City discharged many of its chronic patients to the streets during

Table 1.1. New York City Shelter Survey—Most Recent Year of Discharge from Psychiatric Institution

Year(s)	Number	Percentage
1981	13	28.3
1980	9	19.6
1979	6	13.0
1978	1	2.2
1977	3	6.5
1972–1976	9	19.5
1961–1971	5	10.9
Totals	46	100.0

(From Crystal S. Chronic and situational dependency: long term residents in a shelter for men. New York: NYC Human Resources Administration, May 1982, p. 23. Reprinted with permission.)

the past twenty years. It became an underutilized facility with empty buildings. At the same time, the government of New York City lacked shelter space for the growing number of homeless persons. Logic prevailed, and the state leased the empty space to the city for a nominal sum. Now this city shelter, previously part of the state mental hospital system, houses in substantial number the same people who were previously wards of the State.[37]

THE NEW HOMELESS

The recent prolonged recession left unemployed many people who previously held borderline jobs. A residuum is on the streets and makes up a significant although uncertain number of the homeless.[30,38] An aggravating factor is the chronic problem of high unemployment among black youths and other minority-group members.[13]

Estimates of numbers are weak and their application questionable on a national basis. The most dependable is a thorough analysis carried out at the Keener Shelter in New York City by the Human Resources Administration. Thirty-eight percent of the men who had been at the shelter for two or more months cited joblessness as their reason.

> It is important to note that being "unproductive" members of society is a new status for a large proportion of the homeless. Many men and women speak of past employment as clerks, dishwashers, factory workers, domestics, and various other unskilled occupations . . .[37]

Alienation from family was a significant element as well, indicated as a factor by 28 percent in the Keener study. (See Table 1.2.)

HOMELESS YOUTH

Children and adolescents on the street are often ignored when considering the problem of homelessness. They should be included; and while their health status is probably better than that of older homeless men and women, they are subject to trauma, venereal disease, and psychiatric illness. According to a congressional study released in 1982, there were between 250,000 and 500,000 homeless youths in the United States.[7] Analyses from Boston, Albany, Binghamton, and Buffalo provide support for this rough figure.[39,40] Many of these young people are

Table 1.2. Reason for Admission to Keener

Reason	Number	Percentage
Lost job	48	38.1
Can't stay with family or friend	36	28.6
Want to get off the street	29	23.0
Eviction	23	18.3
Drinking	11	8.7
Hospital discharge	4	3.2
Mugged	4	3.2
Other	45	35.9

Multiple responses were tabulated so percentages total more than 100.

(Adapted from Crystal S. Chronic and situational dependency: long term residents in a shelter for men. New York: NYC Human Resources Administration, May 1982, p. 9. Cited with permission.)

alienated from their families. A considerable proportion were discharged from foster care by superannuation, with no skills and no place to live.[41]

HOMELESS WOMEN

"Bag lady" is an epithet of recent vintage. Until perhaps the mid 1970s, comments on or studies of the homeless population were concerned with men only. We note now a considerable but uncertain number of women in shelters or other locations. Best estimates are that women make up 20 percent or more of the total.[13,26,27,42] Explanations for this development include the deinstitutionalization process; the fact that older women compete poorly in the job market; the reality that they earned salaries lower than men when employed and therefore had less opportunity to establish financial security; the loss of inexpensive housing to urban renewal; singleness or alienation from family; and flight from an abusive spouse.

Homeless women suffer the ills of their male counterparts, as well as conditions specific to the female sex. They are more likely to develop peripheral vascular disease and its consequences because of a sex-borne tendency to varicose veins and venous insufficiency. Bag ladies on the street with massively swollen legs wrapped in rags are a well-known sight. They are more easily victimized and subject to assault. There appears to be a high index of severe emotional disorders in these women. This finding may be factitious, however, because the homeless lifestyle in itself produces emotional reactions that are bizarre.

> To be hungry, cold, deprived of sleep, and socially isolated for even a short period can be mentally and physically wearing. The symptoms of those with mental disabilities are easily exacerbated on the streets. . . . For those who were spared mental illness before they became homeless, the daily stresses of a marginal survival can be highly disorienting . . .[37]

SINGLE-ROOM-OCCUPANCY (SRO) RESIDENTS

Conversion of rental housing to condominiums and cooperatives, known as *gentrification*,[38] has become a compelling financial attraction to real estate interests.[43] As gentrification moves forward, people living in SROs or other inexpensive housing on marginal incomes are the first to be displaced. The street is often the next stop, and then, for some, the shelter system. A 1982 study of new shelter residents in New York City revealed that 61 of 617 men interviewed had spent the previous night in a single-room-occupancy hotel.[33] This phenomenon of displacement has been taking place for more than a decade in New York City.

THE STORY OF THE GREENWICH HOTEL: A PARADIGM OF GENTRIFICATION

The Greenwich Hotel, as it was called in the late 1960s and early 1970s, occupied an eight-story structure in the midst of the entertainment area of Manhattan's Greenwich Village. The surrounding district is occupied largely by middle-class families. It was constructed in 1893 for poor, single, working men.[44] (See Figure 1.1.) Theodore Dreiser is said to have lived in the building, then known as the Mills Hotel No. 1, while he was writing *Sister Carrie*.

In the 1930s the occupants were aged victims of the depression. (See Figure 1.2.)

By the late 1960s it had become a giant SRO, or "welfare hotel." The eight floors of the building had been converted into 1400 cubicles,

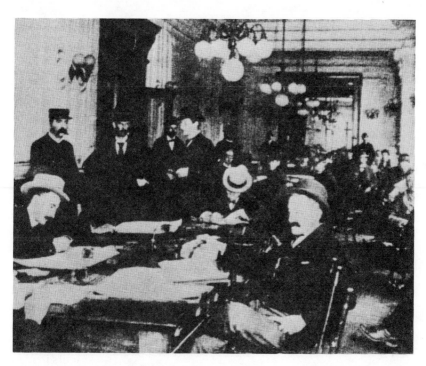

Figure 1.1. The Hotel Interior, 1897 (From Brickner, PW, Kaufman, A. Case finding of heart disease in homeless men. Bulletin of the New York Academy of Medicine, Second Series, Vol. 49, No. 6, p. 476. Copyright © 1973 by the New York Academy of Medicine. Reprinted with permission.)

measuring five by seven feet. Homeless, destitute men were referred to the hotel by the then Department of Social Services of New York City for placement. At the maximum, 1200 people were in residence.

The men fell into three general categories: chronic alcoholics, heroin addicts, and the elderly. About 20 percent of the hotel population were aged men living a marginal existence on social security payments, periodic employment at menial jobs, or welfare. About 35 percent of the men were chronic alcoholics, usually unemployed and living on welfare. The rest, almost half, were heroin addicts, a number of transvestite homosexuals among them, recently released from prison and referred to the hotel by the social service authorities. These men depended on welfare payments as their only legitimate source of income and preyed upon the elderly and alcoholics for money to support their addiction.

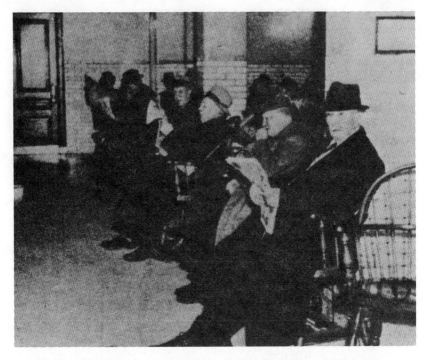

Figure 1.2. The Hotel Interior, 1933 (From Brickner, PW, Kaufman, A. Case finding of heart disease in homeless men. Bulletin of the New York Academy of Medicine, Second Series, Vol. 49, No. 6, p. 477. Copyright © 1973 by the New York Academy of Medicine. Reprinted with permission.)

The hotel management attempted to keep these groups separated by floors and room assignments, but access to all floors was easy. Consequently the younger, more aggressive men freely abused the others. At night the hotel became a jungle in which the aged and disabled barricaded themselves in their rooms or were subject to assault.

Most of the men spent their idle hours loitering in front of the building, hustling for change or drugs in the neighborhood, or wandering in the local park. (See Figure 1.3.)

The reaction of community people to the hotel and to the men themselves was predictable. Local merchants felt that the hotel residents created a negative effect on their trade. Burglaries, muggings, and purse snatchings in the area were generally attributed to these men. After a pedestrian was killed by a table thrown off the roof, pressure was placed upon the mayor's office and the Department of Social

Services to stop supporting welfare clients at the hotel, a policy which took effect in May 1971. All residents whose rent was paid by the city were given the addresses of other welfare hotels. The men left; the political agitation abated. The problem was solved by moving it elsewhere. In later years, as other such buildings closed, many of these people were forced into the streets.

The building ownership was taken over by a real estate entrepreneur, and after reconstruction was reopened in the mid-1970s as a condominium called the Atrium. (See Figure 1.4.)

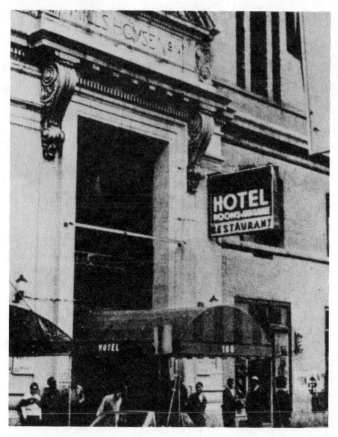

Figure 1.3. The Hotel, Street Scene, 1971 (From Brickner, PW, Kaufman, A. Case finding of heart disease in homeless men. Bulletin of the New York Academy of Medicine, Second Series, Vol. 49, No. 6, p. 479. Copyright © 1973 by the New York Academy of Medicine. Reprinted with permission of the copyright holder and photographer.)

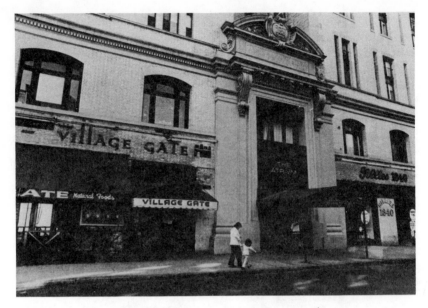

Figure 1.4. The Atrium, Photograph of the Conversion, 1983 (Reprinted with permission of the photographer, Maria Lagudis Lechich.)

INDICES OF DISEASE

Health care for the homeless must deal with the effects of trauma, both major and petty; infestation with scabies and lice, and the skin infections that ensue; peripheral vascular disease, cellulitis, and leg ulcers that stem from the dependent positions in which these men and women keep their legs day after day; alcohol and drug abuse; plus all the standard medical illnesses, including cardiac disease, diabetes mellitus, hypertension, acute and chronic pulmonary disease, and tuberculosis. These matters are reviewed in succeeding chapters. Earlier experience[2,3,45,46] shows that medical problems of SRO residents are similar. (See Table 1.3.)

Clinics were conducted at four SROs in New York City from 1969 through 1972. Seven hundred and forty-three men were seen in a total of 2624 visits. The most common health problems were related to alcohol abuse. Trauma, leg ulcers, cellulitis, and respiratory infection were frequent complaints. Eighty-five men had a history of overt psychosis, and many had been patients in state psychiatric hospitals. Two patients committed suicide in the SROs during this period, and one was murdered.

CHALLENGES

> Since then, whenever in the course of my life I have come across,
> in convents for instance, truly saintly embodiments of practical
> charity, they have generally had the cheerful, practical, brusque
> and unemotioned air of a busy surgeon, the sort of face in which
> one can discern no commiseration, no tenderness at the sight of
> suffering humanity, no fear of hurting it, the impassive, unsym-
> pathetic, sublime face of true goodness.[47]

What is the measure of success for people who work in shelters for the
homeless? Often, small improvements in the lives of patients are tri-
umphs. Failure is common, and for health workers the ability to sustain
a sense of satisfaction and purpose is a test of character. Homeless individuals are often alienated, confused, frightened. Their behavior, by
orthodox standards, is frequently self-defeating. For some, disability
appears preferable to good health.

> Patient A.B., a 65-year-old man, was induced to come for treatment
> of a massive leg ulcer due to venous stasis, trauma and neglect.

Table 1.3. Incidence of Medical Diagnosis in Four New York City SROs: 1969–1972

Diagnosis	*Number*	
Acute or chronic alcoholism	160	
Drug use, intravenous or subcutaneous	102	
Psychosis	85	
Trauma	80	
Assaults		32
Accidents		38
Burns		10
Respiratory infections	76	
Active pulmonary tuberculosis	11	
Cardiovascular disease	54	
Leg ulcers, cellulitis	41	
Acute gastrointestinal disease	22	
Seizure disorders	21	
Jaundice or ascites	20	
Insect infestation	20	
Venereal disease	6	
Gonorrhea		4
Primary syphilis		2
Osteomyelitis	2	

The patient had visited the emergency rooms and outpatient departments of local hospitals but had always refused hospital admission and did not keep clinic appointments. The ulcer involved the entire anterior and lateral surface of the left leg below the knee. Exuberant granulation tissue made the circumference three times that of the right leg. When the patient was first seen, purulent, foulsmelling draining was marked, despite any benefits rendered by the maggots found in the lesion.

Treatment lasted for ten months and consisted of warm antiseptic soaks up to five times per week, sterile dressings, and oral antibiotics. Although the patient was persuaded to visit the clinic daily, he often refused soaks and antibiotics. Improvement was slow.

When reepithelialization was almost complete and drainage minimal, the patient refused to return to the clinic. When observed casually by physicians and nurses, the patient would not discuss his leg, which was seen to be reinfected; the newly formed skin had been destroyed, and gross purulent drainage was present.

When last observed, the patient was semicomatose on the floor. The leg was gangrenous. He was removed to the hospital.[45]

In order to fulfill acceptable standards of humane care for homeless people, health services need to be developed. Creation and training of health care teams in shelters serving the homeless is the first essential step in meeting our obligation. Maturity, self-confidence, and life experience are important assets for staff members.

Voluntary agencies, private philanthropies, and government at all levels must accept the appropriate degree of financial responsibility. Hospitals; workers in the fields of medicine, nursing, and social work; and community agencies must plan together to achieve practical results.

REFERENCES

1. Dostoyevsky F. The brothers Karamazov. ML Edition. 382.
2. Sherman MN, Brickner PW, Schwartz M, Viterella C, Wobido S, Vickery C, Garippa J, Crocco J. Tuberculosis in single-room-occupancy hotel residents: a persisting focus of disease. NY Med Quart. 1980; 2:39–41.
3. Glicksman R, Brickner PW, Edwards D. Tuberculosis screening and treatment of New York City homeless people. Ann NY Acad Sci, in press.
4. Tuberculosis–United States, 1983. MMWR. 1984; 33, 412–15.
5. Bahr HM, Caplow T. Old men drunk and sober. New York: NYU Press, 1973:16–17.
6. Blumberg LU, Shipley TE Jr, Moor JO Jr. The skid row man and the skid row status community. Quart J Stud Alc. 1971; 32:909–41.

7. U.S., Congress, House, Committee on Labor, Oversight hearing on runaway and homeless youth programs before the Subcommittee on Human Resources. 97th Cong., 2d sess., 5 May 1982.
8. O'Connor J. Special report: sheltering the homeless in the nation's capital. Hosp & Comm Psych. 1983; 34:853-65.
9. U.S., Congress, House, Committee on Labor, Oversight hearing, testimony by Gonzalez HB; pp. 1-3.
10. U.S., Congress, House, Committee on Banking, Finance and Urban Affairs, Subcommittee on Housing and Community Development, 15 December 1982. Testimony by Hopper K and Baxter E. US Govt Printing Office, Washington DC, 1983; pp. 28-39.
11. Manhattan Bowery Corporation. Shopping bag ladies; homeless women. New York, 1979.
12. Baxter E, Hopper K. Private lives/public spaces: homeless adults on the streets of New York City. New York: Community Service Society, 1981.
13. Main TJ. The homeless of New York. The Public Interest. 1983; 72:3-28.
14. Osander H. A field investigation of homeless men in Stockholm. Acta Psychiatrica Scandinavica–Supplement 281. 1980; 61:3-125.
15. Freeman SJJ, Formo A, Alampur AG, Sommers AF. Psychiatric disorder in a skid-row mission population. Comprehensive Psych. 1979; 20:454-62.
16. Cooke NJ, Grant IWB. Cost to National Health Service of social outcasts with organic disease. Brit Med J. 1975; 2:132-34.
17. Golyakhovsky V. Russian Doctor. New York: St. Martin's/Marek, 1984:114.
18. U.S., Department of Housing and Urban Development, Office of Policy Development and Research, A report to the Secretary on the homeless and emergency shelters. Washington, DC: May 1984.
19. Cohen C, Sokolovsky J. Toward a concept of homelessness among aged men. J Gerontology. 1983; 38:81-89.
20. Cumming E. Prisons, shelters and homeless men. Psych Quart. 1974; 48(4): 496-504.
21. Morgan M. Skid road: an informal portrait of Seattle. New York: Viking Press, 1962.
22. Bogue DJ. Skid row in American cities. Chicago: University of Chicago Community and Family Studies Ctr, 1963.
23. United States Conference of Mayors. Homelessness in America's cities: ten case studies. Washington, DC: June 1984.
24. Robert Wood Johnson Foundation and Pew Memorial Trust. Health care for the homeless program. Princeton, N.J. and Philadelphia, Pa.: Robert Wood Johnson Foundation, 1983.
25. Jones RE. Street people and psychiatry: an introduction. Hosp & Comm Psych. 1983; 34:807-11.
26. Arce AA, Tadlock M, Vergare MJ, Shapiro SH. A psychiatric profile of street people admitted to an emergency shelter. Hosp & Comm Psych. 1983; 34: 812-17.
27. Lipton FR, Sabatini A, Katz SE. Down and out in the city: the homeless mentally ill. Hosp & Comm Psych. 1983; 34:817,821.

28. Reich R, Siegel L. The emergence of the Bowery as a psychiatric dumping ground. Psych Quart. 1973; 50(3):191–201.

29. Crystal S. Chronic and situational dependency: long term residents in a shelter for men. New York: NYC Human Resources Administration, May 1982.

30. Talbott JA. Commentary: the shame of the cities. Hosp & Comm Psych. 1983; 34:773.

31. Segal SP, Aviram V. The mentally ill in community-based sheltered care. New York: John Wiley, 1978.

32. Kramer M, Pollack ES, Redick RW. Mental disorders/suicide. Cambridge, Mass.: Harvard U Press, 1972.

33. U.S., Department of Health, Education and Welfare, Statistical note 113. State trends in resident patients—State and County Mental Hospitals Inpatient Services, 1967–1973, no. [ADM] 75-158.

34. U.S., Department of Health and Human Services and Department of Housing and Urban Development, Report to the Congress. Report on federal efforts to respond to the shelter and basic living needs of chronically mentally ill individuals. Washington DC, Feb 1983.

35. Talbott JA. Psychiatry's agenda for the '80s. JAMA. 1984; 251:2250.

36. Roberts N. Mental health and mental illness. London: Routledge and Kegan Paul, 1967.

37. Baxter E, Hopper K. The new mendicancy: homeless in New York City. Amer J Orthopsych. 1982; 52(3):393–408.

38. Easterbrook G. Housing: examining a media myth. The Atlantic. 1983; 252:10–26.

39. Kaufman N, Harris J. Profile of the homeless in Massachusetts. Prepared for the Governor's Office of Human Resources. Boston: April 28, 1983.

40. Governor's Task Force on the Homeless. Statewide hearings. Executive Chamber. Albany N.Y.: 1983.

41. Citizens' Committee for Children of New York et al. Homeless youth in New York City: nowhere to turn. New York: September 1983.

42. Slavinsky AT, Cousins A. Homeless women. Nursing Outlook. 1982; 30: 358–62.

43. CORO Public Affairs Leadership Training Program. The effects of cooperative and condominium conversions in New York City. New York: CORO Foundation, May 1981.

44. Llewelyn-Davies Associates. Hotels in Greenwich Village: a study of their use by single men. New York: June 1971.

45. Brickner PW, Greenbaum D, Kaufman A, O'Donnell F, O'Brian JT, Scalice R, Scandizzo J, Sullivan T. A clinic for male derelicts. Ann Int Med. 1972; 77:565.

46. Brickner PW, Kaufman A. Heart disease in homeless men. Bull NY Acad Med. 1973; 49:475–84.

47. Proust M. Remembrance of things past. Swann's way (1913). Trans. by C.K.S. Moncrieff and T. Kilmartin. New York: Random House, 1981:89.

2

Chronic Disease Management in the Homeless

Thomas Filardo

> . . . but the great ocean of distress could not be reduced by bailing with teaspoons.[1]

The definition of chronic diseases is subject to much debate, but in this discussion it will mean those disorders that require continuous intervention by the patient/client and monitoring by health care workers in the traditional clinical setting. Omitted here are lengthy illnesses that are not subject to reversal or arrest by any but extraordinary means, such as the chronic leukemias and the several arthridites. Also omitted are those diseases specifically addressed in other chapters of this book: problems that are either the result of alcohol abuse and/or other conditions prevalent in those who live without regular shelter.

The common chronic ailments for which patients seek medical attention are often silent in their earlier and more treatable states. Hypertension, arteriosclerotic cardiovascular disease (ASCVD), chronic obstructive pulmonary disease, and diabetes mellitus are well known to present symptoms only after significant and irreversible damage has occurred or after a medical emergency has arisen. Some studies on the homeless include prevalence rates for some of these diseases and will be discussed. The various studies that focus on homeless individuals present the reader with some difficult comparisons.

Homelessness itself is not subject to narrow definition, as Cohen and Sokolovsky[2] have shown; Levinson[3] also discusses our ambiguous criteria for homelessness, pointing out how until recently all homeless individuals were assumed to be alcoholics. Distinguishing the homeless from the more advantaged relies more on social than medical criteria. "Sleeping rough," or having no place but the streets to sleep, though little less comfortable or appealing than life in a single-room-occupancy hotel (SRO), offers different stresses to homeless men and women. In the broadest sense, homelessness itself might be considered a chronic disease.

HISTORICAL FOCUS

National focus on problems faced by the homeless among us, currently receiving increased media attention, follows more than a century of scattered literature. Much of the early writing comes from England; but during the times of the earliest reports from there, no similar observations are available from the United States. It appears that only the British surveys can offer us historical perspective.

The Elizabethans spoke of rogues and vagabonds; yet not until the Victorian era, under the guidance of Sir Edwin Chadwick, did England realize that good health in the slums served the personal and economic advantage of the upper classes.[1] A similar realization in the United States has come more slowly and makes historical comparison dangerous. More recent studies might be more comparable. Priest[4] in 1970 found great similarity in the populations of the skid row areas of England and the United States.

Mayhew[5] reviewed the condition of London's poor in 1861. He believed that "[t]he prime cause of vagabondism is essentially the non-inculcation of a habit of industry," and that the majority of those without homes were young men, aged fifteen to twenty-five, mostly "physically stout, healthy lads, and certainly not emaciated or sickly." Those he surveyed with assumed accuracy (estimating the total number of vagrants in England and Wales in 1848 to be 1,647,975) were "not remarkable for a love of drink," but suffered often from "tramp-fever and were the means of spreading pestilence about the nation." Their aversion to being washed, he asserted, was responsible for the large cost of their cures, and they served as "one of the main sources from which the criminals of the country are continually recruited and augmented.'' Of 14,772 individuals reported by the government to have sought refuge in the years 1848–1849, many had lung diseases such as bronchitis, asthma, inflammation, and spitting of blood; and others had catarrh and influenza. Though the diagnostic accuracy of those days may have been inferior to our own, it is clear that lung disease was prevalent among the homeless, accounting for 178 of the 475 illnesses recorded.

The attitude that homelessness and moral turpitude were causally related stayed alive for some years. In 1890, for reasons more religious than governmental, William Booth[6] surveyed London's poorest citizens. Although he mentioned few specific disease statistics, he spoke at length of the wretched conditions in which he found the souls he wished to heal with his newly formed Salvation Army. Charles Booth[7] felt that a discussion of drink ''deserved a prominent place'' in understanding the conditions he found among the poor in East London in 1886. His tone is frequently judgmental as he reflects on the factors leading people to the outcast classes. He admitted an inability to count accurately the inmates of common lodging houses and the ''homeless outcasts''; but he noted that the death rate was highest among the very poor. He found the situation of the homeless as inadmissibly unhealthful from the social science perspective as Preston did from the religious.[8]

In 1903 Jack London,[9] living among the destitute in the city whose name he bore, reported the increased incidence of many diseases that were not officially surveyed. He perceived their cause as self-neglect and noted with alarm the ''smug complacency with which the officials looked upon it and rendered judgement.''

Orwell[10] also provided dramatic inside views of life in the slums of London and Paris, enlarging the understanding of this destitute way of life, which has changed little in this century of monumental societal growth.

During the first half of the current century, concerned as it was with wars that dimmed British and American focus on internal affairs, little was published about the homeless. Beginning in the 1960s on both sides of the Atlantic, the men—rarely women—of skid row became a popular focus of medical investigators, who were largely concerned with psychological aspects and with alcohol abuse. Laidlaw[11] had surveyed the common lodging houses of Glasgow in 1956 and noted a higher morbidity rate than in the general population—12 percent of the men had significant physical illnesses, thus increasing their use of medical services.

CONTEMPORARY STUDIES

In 1963, using data from a United States Public Health Service questionnaire, Bogue[12] published an overview of skid rows in forty-one
American cities, in which he outlined the extent of chronic diseases to
be found among the homeless. One man in ten was found to have a
chronic digestive tract disorder; one in forty, a stomach ulcer; one in
sixteen, hypertension; one in sixteen, heart disease; and one in eleven,
asthma. These were considerably higher prevalence rates than those
reported in the general population at that time.

Despite Levinson's[13] assertion in 1966 that skid rows were to be
found only in America, that same year Scott and colleagues[14] found
skid row people to study in England. This survey of homeless people
who presented themselves at a general practice clinic (an admittedly
select subpopulation of the homeless) appears to be the first attempt
in this century at a longitudinal study of chronic disease management
in the dispossessed. Despite the authors' warning against generaliza-
tion to segments of the homeless population they did not see, the
disease prevalence figures they reported are of interest. Chronic bronchitis was noted in 17.4 percent of their patients, cardiac disease in 5.2
percent, and epilepsy in 4.5 percent. Many of these patients made
several visits to their clinic for treatment. Gaskell[15] again wrote of these
patients and their diagnoses in 1969.

Edwards et al.[16] reported on fifty-one of London's skid row alcoholics in 1966, noting that 16 percent of them had upper gastrointestinal
disease.

In that same year, Olin[17] profiled the skid row syndrome in Canada, noting that epilepsy was found in 8 percent of the men he studied,
gastrointestinal disease in 13 percent, chronic bronchitis in 8.8 percent,
and asthma in 1.3 percent.

In a 1970 editorial, *The Lancet*[18] claimed that the first nationwide attempt to profile the British homeless had been made by the National
Assistance Board "as late as 1966." Women were rarely found among
the homeless, and chronic diseases were "exceptionally common."

Lodge Patch surveyed the London homeless in 1970[19] and 1971[20]
and found that over half of his survey population had a medical complaint in need of attention, with cardiovascular disease occurring in 4
percent, respiratory disease in 9 percent, and epilepsy and other neurological diseases in 11 percent. In 1973 *The Lancet*[21] published an editorial that advised policy development and experimentation to bring
health care to these people.

Brickner et al.[22] studied a welfare hotel population in New York

City in 1972, and in the following year Brickner and Kaufman[23] published a study showing that more than half of these patients suffered from hypertension or arteriosclerotic heart disease.

Blumberg et al.[24] studied Philadelphia's homeless, who again showed a high prevalence of lung disease, hypertension, and ASCVD. Buff et al.,[25] working in a community health center, analyzed one hundred randomly selected charts of SRO residents and again noted a high prevalence of bronchitis, heart disease, and hypertension.

For comparison, hypertension is the most common ambulatory patient diagnosis in the United States (comprising 4.2 percent of all ambulatory patient encounters); ASCVD is the eleventh most common (1.6 percent of all encounters); bronchitis, twelfth (1.6 percent); diabetes, thirteenth (1.6 percent); asthma, eighteenth (1.2 percent); upper gastrointestinal disease, nineteenth (1.1 percent). For the age group over 65, hypertension is again the most common (10.3 percent); ASCVD is second (5.7 percent); diabetes, third (4.0 percent); bronchitis, eleventh (1.5 percent); upper gastrointestinal disease, twelfth (1.5 percent); and cerebrovascular disease, thirteenth (1.4 percent).[26] Strict comparison of these figures to studies of the homeless is difficult, because diagnostic criteria may vary.

Satin et al.[27] has demonstrated that three-dimensional computer mapping of American cities can point to excess mortality from all causes in skid row areas.

Several additional studies in Britain have indicated a similarity of disease patterns between the homeless and those with stable dwellings,[2,28] with increased morbidity in the homeless.[29,31] Mould et al.'s 1978 article[31] was hailed by *The New Scientist* as "the first ever study of mortality patterns among 'the forgotten people.'"

In Sweden, mortality in the homeless was about three times that in the general population during Asander's[32] observation period from 1970 to 1972; Alstrom et al.[33] reported again from Sweden in 1975 that diseases of the gastrointestinal tract and nontuberculous respiratory diseases were each found seven times more frequently in the homeless than in the general population.

At least one study has come from Germany[34] and one from Japan,[35] although the latter is focused solely on hepatitis B.

While the scientific community seems divided in its assessment of the health of those living without permanent shelter, it is enlightening to inquire of the homeless themselves how in need of medical attention they feel to be. Cohen and Sokolovsky[36] found in San Diego that health was of great concern to SRO isolates and that 13 percent (n = 96) rated their health as poor, with older respondents rating their health better than younger ones. Their sample population, divided nearly equally between men and women, had required an average of two hospitalizations for medical diseases in the past ten years, and only 30 percent reported no medically related hospitalizations in that time. For heart disease and hypertension, prevalence rates in these subjects were close to those of the nation as a whole at that time. Eckert[37] demonstrated that the first concern of aged San Diego SRO hotel dwellers was their health. Tissue,[38] studying elderly central-city residents with living conditions that ranged from homeless to home owning, found that 15 percent believed themselves to be in poor health. Shanas et al.[39] surveyed aged persons living in private households and found that, in the United States, 18 percent of those over sixty-five years of age believed themselves to have poor health.

Very few studies appear to have been directed exclusively at homeless women. Slavinsky and Cousins[40] outlined some problems particular to women, and Strasser[41] noted that ten of the thirty-four women she studied had had recent contact with the health care delivery system, though the reasons are not given for these visits. Bogue[12] attested to their rarity in his studies, and Hewetson[30] found that men outnumbered women by twelve to one. Timms[42] did not summarize disease statistics for the homeless girls and women studied. Thus, the prevalence of chronic diseases in the female homeless is not well studied.

The younger homeless represent another poorly studied group of clients with potential chronic diseases. About 40 percent of San Francisco's homeless are military veterans, many of them of the Viet Nam War.[43] "Free clinics" have struggled with the alienated youth of America for some years; they have been reviewed in *The Lancet*[44] and by Schacter and Elliston.[45] Little coordinated epidemiologic study has occurred among them. Holden[46] has set up a special program to help young homeless in London.

ISSUES OF ACCESS

Even in those dense inner-city neighborhoods where health care facilities exist, their presence is no assurance of their being used. Shanks[47] pointed to the suspicion with which the rootless greet medical institutions. Davies[48] documented the largely unmet medical needs of the homeless in England. Hewetson[30] learned that 13 percent of the patients he saw in England's largest shelter had never been registered with a clinic, and that an additional 24 percent were not currently registered with one. Maclean and Naumann[49] found that only 32 percent of hotel residents in Edinburgh were on care lists for a general practitioner, a status guaranteed to all Britons.

What factors dissuade the homeless from seeking health care? In Britain, where such care is provided to any who ask, studies have shown that factors within the health care establishment may be responsible much of the time. Physicians are often reluctant to accept the single homeless; Weir[50] found that more than half the physicians surveyed had refused to accept these patients. That the homeless often come to emergency departments will surprise few who are familiar with the health care systems in America and England; some do so because of the advanced state of their medical condition, and some may do so because of reluctance on the part of physicians to accept them in their offices. Baxter and Hopper[51] pointed to the suspicion with which hospitals are viewed by the homeless, a suspicion often nurtured be memories of or stories about their ineffectiveness and harshness, or because of the bewildering bureaucratic registration and records procedures—aspects of life often shunned by the homeless.

EFFECTIVENESS OF CARE

Bahr[52] has outlined the alienation felt by the homeless. There is growing documentation concerning the interrelatedness of psychological health and primary support systems with physical health. Ehrlich[53] has suggested that the coping mechanisms of SRO occupants leads to denial of physical symptoms. Berkman[54] has shown that social isolation shortens life; Kaplan et al.[55] also studied this phenomenon. Caplan et al.[56] suggested that patient compliance with health care guidelines is related to social support networks.

In addition to these general studies, there is ample evidence in the medical literature to document the ill effects of undue stress on metabolic diseases. Lustman et al.[57] discussed the effects of stress in diabetics; Ornish et al.[58] showed the salubrious effects of stress reduction on ischemic heart disease; and an editorial in *The Lancet*[59] reviewed a great body of literature suggesting that stress aggravates hypertension.

To conclude that the clinical needs of the displaced can be met only after their basic needs for shelter are satisfied is to beg the question. How best to meet the medical needs of these people is an important matter that demands much careful planning. That the homeless population is neither homogeneous nor stable within any city, as has been well documented by Hobfoll et al.[60] in Anchorage, only compounds that difficulty.

DIFFICULTIES WITH CHRONIC CARE

Chronic diseases require constant attention by the patient and regular monitoring by professionals. Given that these might be accomplished with a homeless patient, what forces affect our treatment goals once the patient is back on the streets? Dietary restrictions, imposed frequently for several diseases, are nearly impossible to observe by a patient who has no provisions for cooking and insufficient funds to purchase meals in compliance with guidelines. Soup kitchens, trash bins, and hand-outs do not always yield calorie-controlled or sodium-content-measured portions. Additionally, when some funds might be available for food purchase, the destitute person will likely patronize one of the fast-food restaurants, with their greater tolerance for aberrant dress and behavior, more affordable prices, and more impersonal ambiance. The high sodium and high fat contents of such food have been established.[61]

Surveys concerning the medical status of the homeless point to a high incidence of psychiatric disease among them.[62] Confused patients do not comply with complex medication regimens in the best of circumstances; notes left about the home, pills counted into separate bottles by home health aides or family members do not guarantee sufficient therapy in the best of conditions. With the homeless, profound disorganization of lifestyle militates against even minimal adherence to the simplest medication schedules. Cousins[63] has observed this lack of compliance in homeless patients who use an urban shelter. Given a clear mind and a straightforward medicine schedule, the homeless are still apt to have little attachment to the vague tomorrows of their lives, which may be seen, if at all, as another vista of desperation, a struggle not worth the effort. Tomorrow may be seen as a curse, and medicines that do little to improve the immediate situation may be viewed as useless voodoo.

Brickner and Kaufman found in their 1973 study[23] that only about 50 percent of patients kept their clinic appointments; 59 percent kept their emergency referrals; and 14 percent refused direct admission when an ambulance and attendants were dispatched to transport these very sick men to a hospital. They also found that only one quarter of patients stayed with long-term care. Perhaps a fear of forfeiting bed reservations in an SRO or of losing some other vestige of attachment on the streets pulls the homeless away from a day in the clinic or a night in the hospital.

Poverty prevents patients from acquiring medicines on their own, and the welfare system is not easy to manipulate without frequent trials to patience. Where there is money to be spent, the patient's priorities often differ from those of the health care worker, since shelter, food, or, all too often, substances of abuse are to be had. Lacking a watch, the homeless patient finds medication schedules, which are complex for many chronic diseases, difficult to follow. Once medicines are obtained, storage may present a problem. Bottled pills or capsules must be kept dry, and subjecting them to constant motion, as in a pocket or purse, may reduce them to a useless powder. Insulin creates an obvious storage problem, since refrigeration is rarely available to the homeless; in the cold months, freezing is a similar problem, not only for insulin, but for any medication in liquid form. Establishment of a sterile injection site presents another nearly impossible obstacle in street life. Possession of hypodermic syringes adds a risk of significant magnitude in the violent environment of many of the homeless. Any sort of alcohol for skin cleansing might be ingested or confiscated by others. Poor control of diabetes over years in SRO hotels or shelters may lead to blindness and the other secondary effects of this disease, leading inexorably to institutionalization.

BEGINNING SOLUTIONS

Life on the streets presents stressors of a magnitude and complexity that health care professionals can seldom imagine. Yet the diseases prevalent among the homeless are within the competence of most health care personnel to understand.[64]

The American popular media focused public attention on these people[65,66] with coverage of the federal government's 1983 budget discussions. And still people migrate to large urban centers[67] and remain destitute as federal assistance for the poorest declines.[68]

In England, public attention has been drawn to the problem as well, by Timms,[42] Stewart,[69] and Shanks.[70]

Many programs have been established, and many of the previously cited references originated in them. Many are staffed by individuals volunteering in traditional roles,[29] and some experiment with health visitors.[49,71,72] Others have established clinic-like services in SROs or other similar settings.[22,47,73] Shanks provided a good overview of the various large city programs in Great Britain in his 1982 review.[74] Many hospitals have altered their usual practices to accommodate these patients.[75-77] At least one project shows some impressive epidemiologic success with tuberculosis,[78] providing hope for inroads against other diseases usually considered to be more simply managed.

Hawkins[79] reminds us of the necessity of a nonjudgmental approach toward these patients.

COST

Mayhew spoke about the cost of feeding and treating the homeless of his London.[5] Keighley and Williams[80] more recently pointed out the fiscal advantage of early treatment. The cost of treating a diabetic as an outpatient, for example, is a few dollars per week; the cost of hospitalization for complications of this disease is hundreds of dollars per day. But perhaps the greatest cost of failure to provide early medical treatment is the resulting loss of potential: the loss of opportunity for productive and/or self-rewarding lives for those who cannot find homes in nations of wealth.

REFERENCES

1. Gilbert BB. The evolution of national insurance in Great Britain: the origins of the welfare state. London: Michael Joseph, 1966.
2. Cohen CI, Sokolovsky J. Toward a concept of homelessness among aged men. J Gerontology. 1983; 38:81–89.
3. Levinson BM. The homeless man. Psychological Reports. 1965; 17:391–94.
4. Priest RG. A USA–UK comparison. Proc Roy Soc Med. 1970; 63:441–45.
5. Mayhew H. London labour and the London poor. London: Griffin, 1861.
6. Booth W. In darkest England and the way out. Chicago: Charles H. Sergel & Co., 1890.
7. Booth C. Labour and life of the people. Vol. I. London: Williams & Norgate, 1889:591.
8. Preston WC. The bitter cry of outcast London. London: London Congregational Union, 1883.
9. London J. People of the abyss. London: Isbister, 1903.
10. Orwell G. Down and out in Paris and London. London: Victor Gollancz Ltd., 1933.
11. Laidlaw SIA. Glasgow common lodging houses and the people living in them. Glasgow, 1956.
12. Bogue DJ. Skid row in American cities. Chicago: Community and Family Study Center, University of Chicago, 1963.
13. Levinson BM: Subcultural studies of homeless men. Trans NY Acad Sci. 1966; 29:165–82.
14. Scott R, Gaskell PG, Morrell DC. Patients who reside in common lodging-houses. Brit Med J. 1966; 2:1561–64.
15. Gaskell PG. Illnesses of lodging house inmates. Health Bulletin. 1969; 27:13.
16. Edwards G, Williamson V, Hawker A, Hensman C. London's skid row. Lancet. 1966; 1:249–52.
17. Olin JS. "Skid row" syndrome: a medical profile of the chronic drunkenness offender. Canad Med Assn J. 1966; 95:205–14.

18. Homeless men (editorial). Lancet. 1970; 2:138–39.
19. Lodge Patch IC. Homeless men: a London survey. Proc Roy Soc Med. 1970; 63:437–41.
20. Lodge Patch IC. Homeless man in London: demographic findings in a lodging house sample. Brit J Psychiatry. 1971; 118:313–17.
21. Homeless single persons (editorial). Lancet. 1973; 1:1100.
22. Brickner PW, Greenbaum D, Kaufman A, et al. A clinic for male derelicts. Ann Int Med. 1972; 77:565–69.
23. Brickner PW , Kaufman A. Case finding of heart disease in homeless men. Bull NY Acad Med. 1973; 49:475–84.
24. Blumberg L, Shipley TE Jr, Shandler IW. Skid row and its alternatives. Philadelphia: Temple University Press, 1973.
25. Buff DD, Kenny JF, Light D. Health problems of residents in single-room-occupancy hotels. NYS J Med. 1980; 80:2000–05.
26. National Center for Health Statistics—Gagnon R, De Lozier J, McLemore T. The national ambulatory medical care survey, United States, 1979 Summary. U.S., Department of Health and Human Services, Vital and Health Statistics, Series 13, no. 66, pub. no. (PHS) 82-1727. Public Health Service. Washington, DC: US Govt Printing Office, September 1982.
27. Satin KP, Frerichs RR, Sloss EM. Three-dimensional computer mapping of disease in Los Angeles County. Public Health Reports. 1982; 97:470–75.
28. Blackburn MC. A health profile of homeless vs non-homeless families in central London. Health Visitor. 1981; 54:364–65.
29. MacIntyre D. Medical care for the homeless—some experiences in Glasgow. Scot Med J. 1979; 24:240–45.
30. Hewetson J. Homeless people as an at-risk group. Proc Roy Soc Med. 1975; 68:9–13.
31. Mould R, Wrighton K, Pickup D. Down and out in London and Liverpool. New Scientist. 1978; 77:642–43.
32. Åsander H. A field investigation of homeless men in Stockholm: a socio-psychiatric and clinical follow-up study. Acta Psych Scand. 1980; 61(suppl 281):1–25.
33. Alstrom CH, Lindelius R, Salum I. Mortality among homeless men. Br J Addict. 1975; 70:245–52.
34. Langmann R. [Problems of the homeless from a medical viewpoint]. Oeff Gesundheitswes. 1967; 29:306–12.
35. Monna K, Kawa M, Asai H, et al. Hepatitis B virus and alcoholic liver damage in the Airin district (Osaka's skid row area). Gastroenterologica Japonica. 1980; 15:160–66.
36. Cohen CI, Sokolovsky J. Health-seeking behavior and social networks of the aged living in single-room-occupancy hotels. J Amer Geriatrics Soc. 1979; 27:270–78.
37. Eckert JK. Health status, adjustments and social supports of older people living in center city hotels. Presented at the annual meeting of the Gerontological Society, San Francisco, November 1977.

38. Tissue T. Old age, poverty and the central city. Internat J of Aging and Human Develop. 1971; 2:235–48.
39. Shanas E, Townsend P, Wedderburn D, Friis H, Milhøj P, Stehouwer J. Old people in three industrial societies. New York: Atherton Press, 1968.
40. Slavinsky AT, Cousins A. Homeless women. Nursing Outlook. 1982; 30: 358–62.
41. Strasser JA. Urban transient women. Amer J Nursing. 1978; 78:2076–79.
42. Timms N: Rootless in the city. London: Bedford Square Press, 1968.
43. Reser P: Point man for Viet vets. Mother Jones. 1983; 8:60.
44. America's free clinics—alive and well (news item). Lancet. 1982; 1:1297.
45. Schacter LP, Elliston EP. Medical care in a free community clinic. JAMA. 1977; 237:1848–51.
46. Holden HM. Medical care of homeless and rootless young people. Brit Med J. 1975; 2:446–48.
47. Shanks NJ. Medical provision for the homeless in Manchester. J Roy Coll Gen Pract. 1983; 33:40–43.
48. Davies A. The provision of medical care for the homeless and rootless. London: Campaign for the Homeless and Rootless, 1974.
49. Maclean U, Naumann LM. Primary care for the single homeless: the Edinburgh experiment. Health Bulletin. 1979; 37:6–10.
50. Weir S. Contact before crisis point for those who need care most. Health & Soc Sciences J. 1977; 25:332–33.
51. Baxter E, Hopper K. The new mendicancy: homeless in New York City. Am J Orthopsychiatry. 1982; 52:393–408.
52. Bahr HM. An introduction to disaffiliation. New York: Oxford University Press, 1973.
53. Ehrlich P. St. Louis 'invisible' elderly: needs and characteristics of aged 'single-room-occupancy' downtown hotel residents. St. Louis: Institute of Applied Gerontoloy, St. Louis University, 1976.
54. Berkman L: Social isolation shortens lives. Med World News. Jan 8, 1978: 13.
55. Kaplan BH, Cassel JC, Gore S. Social support and health. Medical Care. 1977; 15(suppl. 47).
56. Caplan RD, Van Harrison R, Wellons RV, French, JR Jr. Social support and patient adherence: experimental and survey findings. Ann Arbor: Survey Research Center, Inst for Soc Research, University of Michigan, 1980.
57. Lustman P, Carney R, Amado H. Acute stress and metabolism in diabetes. Diabetes Care. 1981; 4:568–69.
58. Ornish D, Scherwitz LW, Doody RS, et al. Effects of stress management training and dietary changes in treating ischemic heart disease. JAMA. 1983; 249:54–59.
59. Stress, hypertension and the heart: the adrenaline trilogy (editorial). Lancet. 1982; 2:1440–41.
60. Hobfoll SE, Kelso D, Peterson WJ. The Anchorage skid row. J Studies on Alcohol. 1980; 41:94–99.

61. Young EA, Brennan EH, Irving GL. More perspectives on fast foods. Med Times. 1979; 107:23–30.
62. Leopoldt H, Lynch B. Homeless men in Oxford-1. Nursing Times. 1981; 77:53–56.
63. Cousins AL. Profile of homeless men and women using an urban shelter. J Emerg Nursing. 1983; 9:133–37.
64. Rosenblatt RA, Cherkin DC, Schneeweiss R, Hart LG. The content of ambulatory medical care in the United States: an interdisciplinary comparison. N Engl J Med. 1983; 309:892–97.
65. Easterbrook G. Housing: examining a media myth. The Atlantic. 1983; 252:10ff.
66. Alter J, Stille A, Doherty S. Homeless in America. Newsweek. Jan 2, 1984: 20–29.
67. Jongino JR. Going home: aged return migration in the US, 1965–70. J Gerontology. 1979; 34:736–45.
68. U.S., General Accounting Office. Evaluation of AFDC changes: initial analysis. PEMD-84-6, PSGPO, 1984.
69. Stewart J. Vagrancy and the welfare state. Manchester: Manchester University Press, 1974.
70. Shanks NJ. Care of homeless people, part I. Update. 1981; 23:1197–1202.
71. Fisher E. Homeless families: a scheme of notification to ensure effective care. Nursing Times. 1980; 76:77–80.
72. 'Duchess of the Deuce' helps Phoenix down-and-outs (news item). Am J Nursing. 1981; 8:1529–30.
73. Sr Angela. Rootless and homeless men in Aberdeen. Health Bulletin. 1980; 38:75–76.
74. Shanks NJ. Medical care for the homeless. Brit Med J. 1982; 284:1679–80.
75. Friedman E. On the street: hospitals wrestle with the problem of homeless patients. Hospitals. 1983; 57:97–105.
76. Maitra AK. Dealing with the disadvantaged single homeless: are we doing enough? Public Health. 1982; 96:141–44.
77. Gilpatrick EE. On any avenue. J Psych Nursing and Mental Health Services. 1979; 17:27–30.
78. Shanks NJ, Carroll KB. Improving the identification rate of pulmonary tuberculosis among inmates of common lodging houses. J Epidemiol Comm Health. 1982; 36:130–32.
79. Hawkins R. No way to treat a tramp. Nursing Mirror. 1979; 148:12.
80. Keighley RAS, Williams HM. Cost to NHS of social outcasts with organic disease. Brit Med J. 1975; 2:389.

PART II

MEDICAL DISORDERS

3

Infestations: Scabies and Lice

Richard W. Green

In 1983 the two most common diagnoses in the emergency room of a large San Francisco hospital were scabies and pediculosis (lice).[1] Whereas parasitic skin infestations might be an unusual event in the hospital of a small town where full employment reigns, in an economically (and socially) depressed area with many homeless and poor people, diseases of this type are common. There are other insects that attack the homeless, such as fleas and bedbugs, but they are not parasites to humans, the morbidity is much less, and the treatment is much simpler.

Lice and scabies have been around since biblical times and have played a significant role in culture and history. Because lice were such a problem in Europe, many men and women in high society shaved their heads and donned wigs. Unfortunately, this offered little relief, since the lice and nits readily invaded the wigs and moved freely back to the scalp.[2]

During the 1680s the Turkish army rampaged through Western Europe, meeting little resistance until it reached the well-fortified city of Vienna. While laying siege to the city, a lice-borne epidemic erupted, killing many soldiers and their leaders. The weakened army was forced to retreat and Vienna was saved. But for the presence of lice, Turkish might be spoken in Paris today.[2] Scabies and pediculosis wreaked havoc in the trenches of World Wars I and II and, more recently, troubled the Argentine troops serving in the Falklands.

SCABIES

Scabies is caused by a highly contagious parasite and manifests clinically as an intensely itchy, cutaneous disease. In recent years the incidence of this disease has increased in most parts of the world, including the United States. Because physicians are not required to report cases of scabies to the public health authorities, true figures of the national increase of scabies infestation are not available.[3] However, the increased sales of scabicides indicate a rise in the incidence of scabies and/or pediculosis (scabicides are also pediculicides). For the twelve-month period ending December 1980, the National Disease and Therapeutic Index reported approximately 655,000 patient visits for scabies. This represents an elevenfold increase over the 1970 figure, and a twofold increase over the 1974 estimate.[4] Figures from the social hygiene clinics of the New York City Department of Health show a 117.3 percent increase in the incidence of scabies from 1978 (214 cases) to 1982 (465 cases).[3]

Although scabies is not a life-threatening disease, the complications from secondary infection can be serious. These include internal abscesses, pyogenic pneumonia, septicemia, and secondary impetigo with acute glomerulonephritis. The itching caused by scabies can be extreme and can prevent sleep, efficiency, and employment.

Human scabies is caused by the mite *Sarcoptes scabiei var. hominis*, an arthropod of the order Acarina. (See Figure 3.1.) The mite is host specific, and mites that infest other mammals will not survive for an extended period on human skin. The mite is eyeless, oval, and translucent, with brown spines and bristles, and eight short legs. The male mite is 1.2 mm in length while the adult female, the most commonly encountered organism, is 0.3 mm. The female can walk on the skin at a rate of 2½ cm per minute.[4] After copulation with a male mite on the skin surface, the fertilized female excavates a sloping burrow in the stratum corneum (the dead horny cell layer of the epidermis).[5] Within this blind tunnel, which may be 1 cm long, the female lays ten to twenty-five eggs before dying. The eggs hatch within three to four days, and the emerging larvae mature on the skin surface in fourteen to seventeen days after passing through larval and nymphal stages. The male of the species has a shorter life span than the female, lives ex-

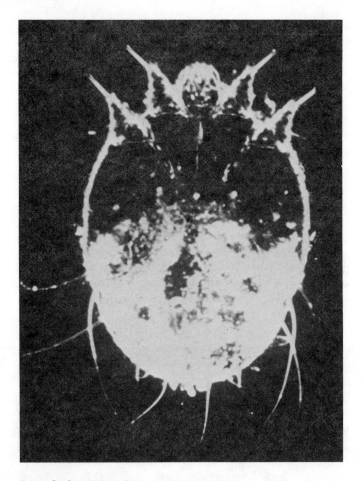

Figure 3.1. Scabies Mite (Reprinted with permission of Reed and Carnrick Pharmaceuticals.)

clusively on the surface of the skin, and plays a lesser role in the disease process.

The skin disease associated with scabies is considered to be a cell-mediated hypersensitivity response to the mite or its products.[5] For the first four to six weeks after an infestation, there may be no clinical symptoms. After this host sensitization period, the characteristic skin lesions appear together with the intense itching. Once the host has been sensitized, future infestations with scabies will result in the characteristic eruption and itching within as short a period as twenty-four hours.[3]

Failure to develop an allergic reaction to the mite or its products can result in a condition called Norwegian or crusted scabies. (See Figure 3.2.) Victims of this condition frequently have Down's syndrome or are otherwise mentally deficient or immunocompromised, due either to a primary immune disorder or the use of immunosuppressive drugs. They do not itch and therefore do not scratch and destroy or dislodge the mites or their eggs. Eleven is the average number of mites present in a patient with ordinary human scabies,[3] whereas patients with Norwegian scabies may have upwards of two million mites and are highly contagious.

Signs and Symptoms

The main symptom of scabies is intense itching, which usually increases in severity as the patient tries to sleep. Although the increased itching at night is not clearly understood, several hypotheses have been suggested. One theory is that the mites' activity increases with the warmer

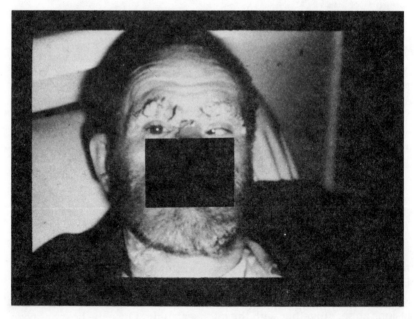

Figure 3.2. Norwegian Scabies Victim (Reprinted with permission of New York University School of Medicine, Department of Dermatology.)

skin temperature caused by bedding and night clothes. Another theory is that the mite may be nocturnally active because of light sensitivity.[4] The transparency of the organism would suggest that possibility. The itch of scabies is of such intensity that the scratching often causes bleeding. This is unusual with other dermatoses. Historically, bloodied sheets, pajamas, or underwear strongly suggest scabies.[4]

The physical signs of scabies consist of a rash with minute blisters, excoriations, and small, linear crusts. These lesions are in different stages of development in each patient. The characteristic lesion is the burrow (the small, linear crust), which is wavy, threadlike, and measures 1 to 10 mm in length. (See Figure 3.3.) The mites tend to colonize on certain areas of the skin regardless of the site of the original contact.[5] Common locations are the interdigital webbing of the hands and the wrists, axillae, waist, lower buttocks, umbilicus, feet, and ankles. In women the breasts are frequently involved. In men, the penis and scrotum are affected. The back, chest, and head are usually spared in adults, but in infants all skin surfaces are susceptible. Secondary infections due to scratching are not uncommon. Generalized urticaria (hives) has been reported by Witkowski and Parish.[6]

Atypical forms of scabies exist, although they are uncommon. Norwegian scabies must be considered in the mentally and physically disabled, for whom itching is not a prominent symptom.

"Scabies in the clean," or "scabies in the cultivated," occurs in people who are obsessed with cleanliness and bathe very often. They literally wash away many of the mites and their products. Findings may be minimal, with burrows found in only 7 percent of cases.

The use of topical corticosteroids masks or alters the usual skin findings of scabies incognito.[7] While the symptoms may be minimal, it is still contagious. It is sometimes misdiagnosed as impetigo or a superficial fungus infection.

Nodular scabies is still another form. Patients afflicted with this condition develop indurated skin-colored or pigmented pruritic nodules, primarily on covered parts of the body (male genitalia, groin, or axillae); the nodules may persist for more than a year despite therapy. Mites are seldom demonstrated in nodules present for more than one month.

Scabies has recently been reported in a patient with *Pneumocystis carinii* pneumonia,[8] a type of pneumonia frequently found in patients with acquired immune deficiency syndrome (AIDS). While scabies has not been reported in patients with AIDS, it is reasonable to assume that if they contract scabies, it would be in a virulent form.

Another form of scabies is the so-called "animal transmitted

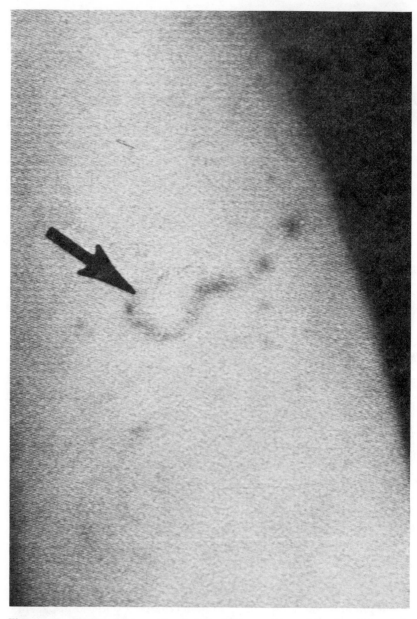

Figure 3.3. Scabies Burrow (Reprinted with permission of Reed and Carnrick Pharmaceuticals.)

scabies." Although persons may be infested with mites from a variety of domestic animals, including poultry, dogs (usually puppies) are the major source.[7] These mites are morphologically similar to the human mite but differ in their biological behavior. They do not burrow or breed in humans, and consequently the condition is limited to the life span of the mites (three to four weeks) unless the patient is reinfested. This form of scabies in man differs from human scabies in its greater ease of transmission, a shorter incubation period, and a different distribution pattern. It is usually less itchy, which could be attributed to the inability of these mites to form burrows. Man is usually parasitized by petting or touching the animal. In the dog the external ear is the most common site of infection.[7] Since this form of scabies does not reproduce itself, specific therapy is not necessary but may be given to relieve the itching. The host animal should be treated.

Other types of nonburrowing mites found in plants, foods, and animals that affect humans were recently reviewed by Shelley et al.[9] These patients had a strongly positive mite antigen skin test.

Diagnosis

Stokes called a scabies "at once the easiest, and the most difficult diagnosis in dermatology."[10] Scabies has also been called the "great imitator," a term used in the past for syphilis. The diagnosis is, however, frequently easy; and it can be presumed if the patient has a skin eruption with crusts, excoriations, and burrows in the commonly involved areas, intense nocturnal itching, and a history of possible contact with other "itchy" people. The definitive diagnosis requires the identification of the mite, fecal pellets (scybala), or the eggs. Burrows, where the mites are most readily found, are present in over 95 percent of patients with the disease. The best places to find the burrows include the interdigital areas of the hands (see Figure 3.4), as well as the wrists, elbows, sides of hands, feet, and ankles.[4] Burrows can be observed more readily with the following techniques:

1. The application of mineral oil to the affected area alters the refractive index of the stratum corneum and allows better visibility.

2. Liquid tetracycline is applied to areas where burrows are usually found. After several minutes the area is wiped with alcohol. The tetracycline penetrates any areas of the stratum corneum that are disrupted, i.e., the burrow. A portable Woods lamp will fluoresce the burrows a yellow-grey color. This method has an advantage over the ink test (see

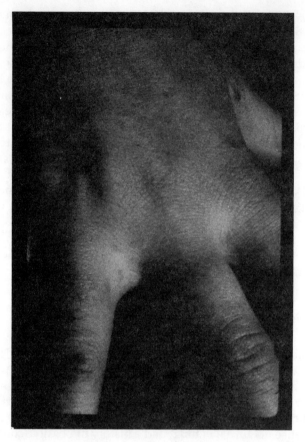

Figure 3.4. Scabies Infestation at Typical Site (Reprinted with permission of Reed and Carnrick Pharmaceuticals.)

below) in that the relatively colorless tetracycline can be applied over large areas.[11]

3. The ink test, using ordinary fountain-pen ink, will, in a like manner, penetrate the burrow; and it is simpler to use. The excess ink is wiped away and a ragged line (the burrow) remains.

The mites and their products can usually be identified once the burrows are found. The simplest method is an epidermal shave biopsy.[12] The lesion is superficially shaved or scraped with a #15 scalpel blade after applying immersion oil or mineral oil to the skin. The oil holds the debris together so that it can be transferred to a glass slide. A coverslip is applied and the debris is examined under low power magnification.

A deeper skin biopsy is also useful in demonstrating the mite; however, it is usually done only when the index of suspicion is high and the other techniques have failed to disclose the organisms. It is a relatively costly technique.

Treatment

The most widely used agent for the treatment of scabies in this country is gamma benzene hexachloride (GBHC, lindane, GBH®, Kwell®). It is both an ectoparasiticide and ovacide and is available as a 1 percent creme, lotion, and shampoo, the latter used primarily for the treatment of pediculosis. The lotion, easier to use than the creme, is applied from the neck to the toes, with special emphasis at the sites of predilection. It is left on for six to eight hours and then washed off thoroughly. Approximately one ounce of lotion is required to cover the trunk and extremities of an average adult.[13] If the hands are washed after the medication has been applied, it should be reapplied to them. One application has a cure rate of 96–98 percent.[4] A second application can be given four to seven days later if necessary.

The clothes the person wore the preceding day and the bed linens are washed in hot water (the mites cannot survive temperatures higher than 120°F for more than five minutes)[14] or set aside for three days. The organism is an obligate parasite of humans and will exist for only two to three days when away from human skin.[15] Hence, clothes worn prior to three days before treatment would not have living mites and would be safe to wear.

GBHC can cause central nervous system (CNS) toxicity when the drug is misused; when used appropriately, however, toxicity has never been proven.[3]

To reduce GBHC's real or imagined toxicity, Solomon[16] advises:

1. avoiding a hot, soapy bath, which increases absorption of the drug, prior to treatment;
2. applying the medication for the shortest period of time necessary to cure scabies;
3. discouraging repeated usage and use of anything but the lowest possible effective concentration of the medication.

Rasmussen[17] is concerned about toxic reactions that have occurred following misuse of GBHC and advises additional therapeutic recommendations as follows:

1. Tell *all* your patients that Kwell can be toxic when misused. Better to hear it from you than from a pharmacist, friend, or health columnist.
2. Write "no refills" on all prescriptions and use just enough for the patient and contacts.
3. Never re-treat within one week, and tell your patients why. The fear of a convulsion will go a long way toward ensuring proper compliance.
4. Consider dispensing the drug yourself or recommending a pharmacy that knows your personal concern about Kwell.[17]

Because of potential toxicity of Kwell in infants and children, 5 percent sulfur in petrolatum has been recommended. Another scabicide, crotamiton, is also effective. However, Rasmussen[17] states that "the alternate agents suggested as safer for infants and children are nearly unknown quantities: their efficacy is questionable and toxicology unstudied (or distressingly similar to the CNS toxicity of lindane)."

Although GBHC is lethal to the mites and their eggs, itching can persist for one to two weeks until the mite antigens are sloughed off. A moisturizing creme may be helpful after completion of antiscabietic therapy. Topical corticosteroids are contraindicated prior to therapy but may be useful in patients who continue to have pruritus following antiscabietic therapy. The GBHC lotion itself can cause skin irritation, and its repeated use should be considered as a cause of persistent itching.

Once scabies is diagnosed, all the close personal contacts and household members of the infested individual should be treated at the same time. Such contacts may be asymptomatic because of the four to six week incubation period, but they must be treated nonetheless.

PEDICULOSIS

A forty-year-old man, who appears much older, shuffles into the emergency room in a local hospital in the poorer section of town. He is nervous, shaky, and relates to the intern that he cannot sleep, feels awful, and itches all over. The young intern, recently graduated from medical school, quite astutely believes his new patient is an alcoholic who has come to the hospital for a few days of rest and good (sic) food.

The history confirms moderate to heavy wine and whiskey consumption, homelessness, and hunger. The physical examination reveals signs of poor nutrition, a nonspecific rash with excoriations on the upper trunk, and a low-grade fever. The tentative diagnosis is chronic alcoholism, malnutrition, and probable early cirrhosis of the liver. The intern turns to hand the patient his tattered wool shirt only to find multiple crawling things at the collar line and seams. Reexamination of the patient reveals a few nits on the hairs of his chest and many nits on the fibers of his clothing. The diagnosis is changed to *Pediculus humanus corporis*, or body lice, which explains the rash, the itching, and probably accounts for the low-grade fever. While he may indeed have liver pathology, his parasitic infestation is his primary medical problem at this time.

There are three kinds of pediculi, commonly known as lice: *Pediculus humanus capitis*, the head louse (see Figure 3.5); *Pediculus humanus corporis*, the body louse; *Phthirus pubis*, the crab or pubic louse. All are ectoparasites, with humans as their only hosts. They are small, dorsoventrally flattened, wingless insects, greyish-white in color and 0.8 to 4.0 mm in length. The body has three parts: an angular, ovoid head; a fused thorax; and a segmented abdomen. These distinctions are more difficult to see in the crab louse because of its more oval shape and smaller size. (See Figure 3.6.) Each louse has a pair of simple, lateral eyes and a pair of short antennae. Six pairs of hooklets surround the mouth at the forehead and are used to grab onto the skin during feeding. In front of the oral opening is a piercing extension, or proboscis, with a central duct through which salivary secretions are introduced into the wound. These secretions have an anticoagulant that facilitates withdrawal of blood. The thorax has three pairs of short, stout legs that end in sharp, curved claws. The claws permit the louse to grasp and hold firmly onto the hair or clothing. The presence of six legs characterizes the louse as an insect. The abdomen contains the digestive tract and reproductive organs.

The entire life cycle of lice is completed on the host, although the body louse spends most of its time on the fibers of the host's clothing. After reaching maturity the impregnated female lays eggs at the rate of approximately six every twenty-four hours.[2] She attaches the ova firmly to the hair shaft (see Figure 3.7) or clothing fibers with a secretion that bonds the egg to the hair or clothing fiber. The egg, together with the cement, is called a nit; nits are 0.6 to 1.0 mm in length.

In five to ten days the eggs hatch, and the larvae quickly mature into adults. Although lice spend their entire life cycle on or close to human skin and can live without feeding for two to ten days,[2] the nits can survive for up to thirty-five days. If a nit is found close to the skin

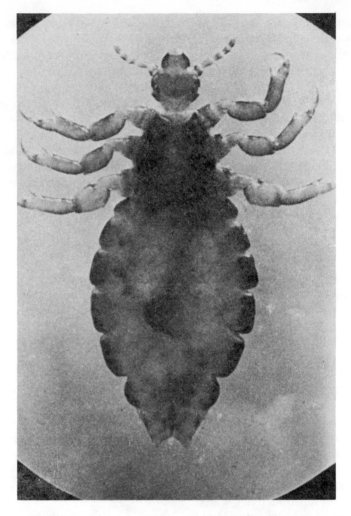

Figure 3.5. Head Louse (Reprinted with permission of Reed and Carnrick Pharmaceuticals.)

surface, it is probably a living nit unless the patient has been treated. If the nit is two or more mm away from the skin surface, it is more than ten days old and unlikely to be viable. In order to hatch, a nit requires a temperature of over 22°C (72°F)[2,18] and needs to be within 1 to 2 mm of the skin surface.

All three kinds of lice are dependent on their host for food. They feed approximately five times a day by sucking blood for extended periods; unlike ticks, however, they apparently do not become engorged. Feeding time averages from thirty-five to forty-five minutes, and digestion takes about four hours.[2]

Nymphs and adult lice are active travelers. Body and head lice travel by grasping hairs and clothing fibers, swinging like Tarzan. This mobility allows them to pass readily from host to host. However, when

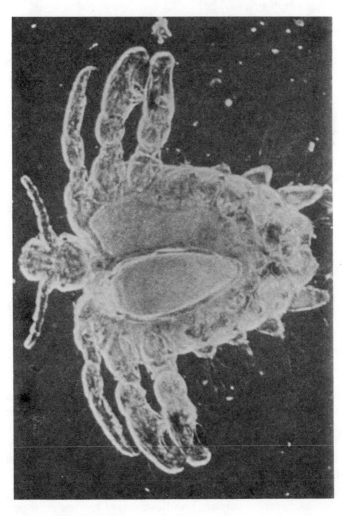

Figure 3.6. Crab Louse (Reprinted with permission of Reed and Carnrick Pharmaceuticals.)

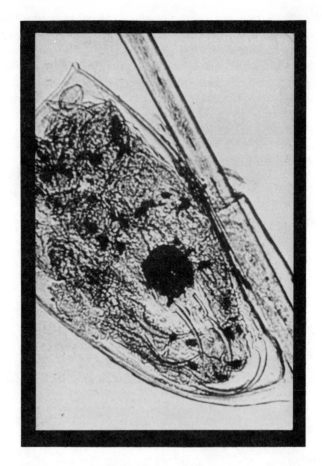

Figure 3.7. Nit on Hair Shaft (Reprinted with permission of Reed and Carnrick Pharmaceuticals.)

clothing is removed from a person with body lice, the lice remain motionless, clustered around the seam. (See Figure 3.8.) When head lice are seen, they are usually traveling about in the hair. The less athletic crab louse utilizes hairs only for the egg laying/nit building process. Crab lice are usually dug into the outer layer of skin and appear to be motionless.

Clinical characteristics of lice infestations are as follows:

Pediculus humanus capitis: The head louse causes erythematous, papular, and crusted lesions in the scalp, the back of the neck, and the upper shoulders. Scratching and secondary inflammation can lead to an oozing dermatitis, matted hair, and bacterial infection. Saliva injected by the lice can cause a low-grade fever, muscular aches, and occasional swelling of the cervical glands. On physical examination, the adult lice are difficult to see, but numerous nits, firmly cemented to the hair, are readily detectable. The nits are easily differentiated from seborrheic scales and hair casts, which can be moved along the shaft of the hair.[2] The nits are visible to the naked eye and the diagnosis may be made on that basis. Rapid examination of large groups of people is facilitated by Woods light examination of the scalp.[18] Infested hair becomes fluorescent under ultraviolet light.

Pediculus humanus corporis: The body louse, the largest of the species,

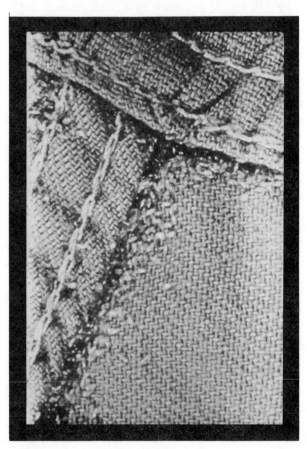

Figure 3.8. Body Lice on Clothing (Reprinted with permission of Reed and Carnrick Pharmaceuticals.)

lives and can readily be seen in the clothing of the host, although occasionally it can be observed feeding. Its saliva causes an itchy, erythematous, papular rash. (See Figure 3.9.) When infestation is heavy and nutrition poor, chills, fever, and muscular aches can result. As the name suggests, the clinical manifestations are primarily confined to the body, i.e., chest, abdomen, and upper back. The extremities are infrequently involved, possibly due to the lack of seams in the clothing in those areas. The infestation primarily affects men because of their body hair.

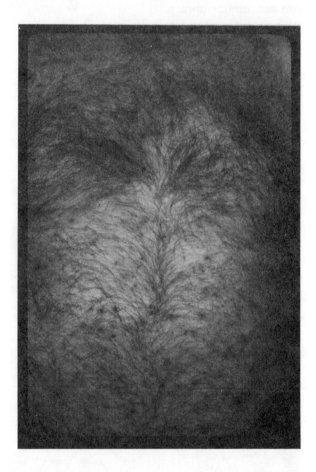

Figure 3.9. Body Lice Infestation (Reprinted with permission of New York University School of Medicine, Department of Dermatology.)

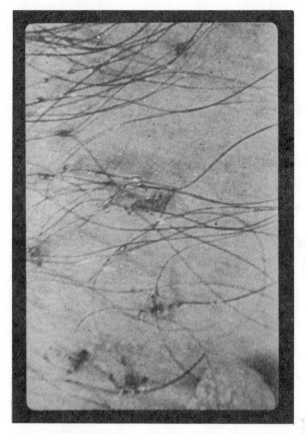

Figure 3.10. Crab Lice Infestation (Reprinted with permission of Reed and Carnrick Pharmaceuticals.)

Phthirus pubis: As the name suggests, this louse mainly affects the pubic area; the thighs, lower abdomen, and axillae are frequently infested as well. (See Figure 3.10.) Other hairy areas, including the eyelids, can be involved. The scalp is spared. Pubic lice, the smallest of the three, are difficult to spot but can easily be seen with the aid of a magnifying lens. They hold on to the skin tenaciously as one tries to remove them with a forceps. The nits are seen wherever lice are, although, in the axillae, nits are frequently seen but not the lice. Secondary skin infections are less common in *Phthirus pubis*. Itching is the most prominent symptom.

Transmission

Homeless people spread body lice by exchanging clothing, by picking up clothing off the streets, and by lying next to one another in hallways, on park benches, and on sidewalks. Head lice are spread by exchanges of combs, brushes, and headgear, as well as by close physical contact. The head louse is hardier than the body or pubic louse and can live away from its human host for several days.[19] Pubic lice are usually transmitted by sexual contact. This type of lice infestation is less common among the homeless.

Treatment

The treatment of pediculosis utilizes GBHC, the same medication used for scabies. In head lice, GBHC shampoo is used. After one fifteen-minute shampoo, the patient should put on freshly laundered or dry-cleaned clothing and use fresh bed linens. Hats should be dry cleaned or subjected to drying at high heat for twenty minutes. Combs and brushes should be dipped in boiling water or washed in hot water—54.4°C (130°F)—for ten minutes.[20]

Pubic lice are treated with GBHC lotion or shampoo. The medication is applied to all hairy areas but the scalp. Clothing and bed linens should be machine washed and heat dried or laundered and then ironed. Therapeutic failure is usually caused by reinfestation or failure to follow instructions properly.

The treatment of body lice emphasizes the patient's garments and measures to improve the patient's personal hygiene. The patient should be given clean clothing and bedding. All clothing that the patient has worn in the previous three days, which in the homeless usually means whatever he is presently wearing, should be dry cleaned, or machine washed in the hot cycle and ironed. If the patient's clothes are not worth saving, then they should be disposed of in a plastic bag. Plastic gloves should be worn when handling the clothing.[19] If there are nits on the patient, then GBHC lotion should be applied to all hairy areas except the scalp.

As with scabies, itching can persist for one to two weeks after therapy. It is caused by the dead organism or its products, by an irritant reaction to the medication, or, in part, by the persistence of allergic skin hypersensitivity.

Body lice can also transmit the infectious agent that causes relapsing fever and epidemic typhus. In underdeveloped countries such as Pakistan and India, these diseases still occur.

Parasitophobia is not uncommon in the homeless with or without physical evidence of active infestation. It can be troublesome and requires repeated reassurance.

COMMENTS—SCABIES AND LICE

In conclusion, several points are sufficiently worthy to deserve highlight:

1. Although scabies is usually considered a sexually transmitted disease, the primary means of transmission in the homeless is the act of sleeping next to another. Casual intimate contact such as dancing, petting, or holding hands may, however, transmit the disease.

2. While it is important to track down, examine, and treat suspected contacts, there have been many patients with proven scabies whose contacts were not infested.

3. Good hygiene will not prevent scabies, as is shown in hospital outbreaks and the rising incidence in military personnel.[5] However, crowded living conditions, the sharing of sleeping accommodations, and the infrequent laundering of clothes certainly favors its spread.

4. Infants and children acquire scabies from their parents or other children. Fomites, such as upholstered furniture and beds, seem to play a larger role in childhood scabies than they do in the transmission of scabies in adults. Wrestling mats have been known to transmit scabies in teenagers and young adults.

5. It is not necessary to clean carpeting, floors, furniture, or outerwear, since this is a very unlikely source of transmission of adult scabies. Guidelines are less certain in childhood scabies.

6. It should be remembered that scabies and lice can coexist with other itchy or nonitchy skin diseases. The scabies or lice may be cured, but the other skin disease may persist and confuse. Venereal diseases should be considered when diagnosing scabies and lice infestations.

7. The great difficulty in treating lice and scabies in the homeless is that we cannot simultaneously treat all their contacts. Normally if a patient has scabies we treat every contact in the home or institution simultaneously. If a patient has lice, we examine and then, if necessary, treat all the contacts. In the homeless, however, the contacts often cannot be found and, if found, cannot be treated at the same time as the index case. This time gap allows for reinfestation of other contacts as well as the index case.

The homeless, by definition, have temporary shelters or are moving from park bench to deserted storefronts to culverts to ventilation grids in the streets. They sleep next to one another for warmth and social comfort; they share clothing, and pick up clothing off the street; they share bedding, and their hygiene is frequently nonexistent.

Infestations can be treated successfully and theoretically could be eradicated if all those affected could be treated. Progress in this direction requires the education of health personnel, social workers, hospital administrators, and the staff of shelters for the homeless.

A high index of suspicion of infestations must be maintained, and measures must be taken to improve the sanitary conditions, the overcrowding, and the social attitudes that foster the indifference or resignation of those afflicted.

REFERENCES

1. Kelly J. Personal communication. October 1983.
2. Lice and scabies: from infestation to disinfestation. Kenilworth, N.J.: Reed and Carnrick (no date).
3. Felman Y, Nikitas J. Scabies. Cutis. 1984; 33:266–75.
4. Estes S. The diagnosis and management of scabies. Kenilworth, N.J.: Reed and Carnrick, 1981.
5. Burkhart C. Scabies: an epidemiologic assessment. Ann Intern Med. 1983; 98:498–503.
6. Witkowski JA, Parish LC. Scabies: A cause of generalized urticaria. Cutis. 1984; 33:277–79.
7. Orkin M. Today's scabies. JAMA. 1975; 233:882–85.
8. Miyoshi I, Sonobe H, Taguchi H, Kubonishi I, Kobayashi M. Association of *Pneumocystis Carinii* pneumonia and scabies. JAMA. 1982; 248:1973.
9. Shelley ED, Shelley WB, Pila JF, McDonald SG. The diagnostic challenge of non-burrowing mite bites: *cheyletiella yasquri.* JAMA. 1984; 251:2690–91.
10. Stokes JH. Scabies among the well-to-do. JAMA. 1936; 106:674–78.
11. Dotz W, Berman B. Scabies: an immunologic, diagnostic and therapeutic update. Medical Times. February 1983.
12. Martin W, Wheeler CE Jr. Diagnosis of human scabies by epidermal shave biopsy. J Am Acad Dermatol. 1979; 1:335–37.
13. Orkin M, Epstein E Sr., Naibach HI. Treatment of today's scabies and pediculosis. JAMA. 1976; 236:1136–39.
14. Parish L. Nobody gets scabies anymore. Consultant. May–June 1970:24–26.
15. Estes SA, Aolian L. Survival of *Sarcoptes Scabei* (letter). J Am Acad Dermatol. 1981; 5:243.
16. Solomon LM, Sahrnar L, West DP. Gamma benzene hexachloride toxicity: a review. Arch Derm. 1977; 113:353–57.

17. Rasmussen JE. The problem of lindane. J Am Acad Dermatol. 1981; 5: 507–16.
18. Juranek DD. *Pediculosis capitis* in school children: epidemiologic trends, risk factors, and recommendations for control. In: Orkin M, Naibach HI, eds. Lice infestation update: transmission and treatment. New York: Marcel Dekker, 1983:17–29.
19. Feinstein RJ. Ectoparasitic infections. Dermatology. 1978; 68:30–32.
20. Orkin M, Naibach HI. Treatment of today's pediculosis. In: Orkin M, Naibach HI, eds. Lice infestation update: transmission and treatment. New York: Marcel Dekker, 1983:31–35.

4

Exposure: Thermoregulatory Disorders in the Homeless Patient

Lewis Goldfrank

Physiologic, metabolic, nutritional, neurologic, vasomotor, toxicologic, and psychologic adaptations to the environment are impaired by exposure and thermal stress. The homeless are at particular risk because the world of the street is unprotected from sun, wind, snow, and rain. Some of the resulting problems are well understood, and some are poorly defined. Most involve complex interactions of the aforementioned conditions. Because the homeless often seek health care only when they have a multiplicity of problems, it is difficult to define precisely the etiologic factors responsible for their thermoregulatory emergencies. A basic discussion must include a review of physiologic interactions with the environment. This description will allow for a better understanding of the complex pathologic states precipitated by the inability of the homeless to achieve effective adaptive mechanisms to the environmental extremes of summer and winter.

PHYSIOLOGIC MECHANISMS
OF THERMOREGULATION

The major mechanisms of thermal control are radiation, conduction, convection, respiration, evaporation, and excretion.[1,2] (See Table 4.1.) These mechanisms are balanced by our basal metabolic rate, which usually allows homeostasis to be achieved. Normal body temperature is defined as 98.6°F (37°C). Definitions vary, but a rectal temperature lower than 95°F (35°C) or higher than 100°F (37.8°C) is considered to be abnormal. Many individuals have a set point above or below 98.6°F (37°C), but the homeostatic mechanisms are usually so well developed that there is rarely a variation greater than 1°F (0.6°C) on any particular day. The normal variation usually follows a circadian rhythm, with the lowest body temperature at dawn and the highest at twilight. The extent of thermostability and the presence or absence of a circadian rhythm have never been studied in homeless patients, whose style of life is irregular, but it is well known that the cycles are reversed for those who work from evening until morning.

Conduction of heat is determined by the thermal gradient between the human body and a surface. For example, there is a direct transfer

Table 4.1. Equation Relating Thermal Control Mechanisms to Basal Metabolic Rate

$$S = M \pm C_1 \pm C_2 \pm R_1 \pm R_2 - E_1 - E_2$$

S = Heat storage

M = Basal metabolic rate = 65–85 Kcal/hr, but increases dramatically with any substantial motor activity or exercise.

C_1 = Conduction—The direct transfer of heat to cooler objects or receipt of heat from warmer objects when direct contact is made. Heat transfer is proportional to the thermal gradient.

C_2 = Convection—The transfer of heat is dependent on the wind velocity, humidity, and ambient air temperature.

R_1 = Respiration—Heat loss is the amount needed to warm inhaled air to body temperature or the amount absorbed from the air.

R_2 = Radiation—The transfer of heat to those cooler parts of the environment not in contact with the body, or receipt of heat from external sources.

E_1 = Evaporation—Water is evaporated from the body surface, depending on the temperature, air velocity, and humidity.

E_2 = Excretion—Heat loss from feces and urine.

(From Goldfrank LR, Flomenbaum N, Lewin N, Weisman RS. Nonseasonal Heatstroke. Hospital Physician. 1982; 18(6): 50–70. Copyright © by PW Communications, 1982. Reprinted with permission.)

of heat from the skin to a cold grate or park bench in winter; or from those same heated metals to the body in summer. The mechanism of this heat transfer may be directly responsible for frostbite in winter and a first or second degree burn in summer.

Convection of heat is dependent upon the wind velocity, humidity, and ambient air temperature. The greater the amount of exposed surface area, the greater the thermal stress. The wind-chill factor is a means of interpreting the thermal impact of convection and must be considered a critical parameter for thermal stability in the exposed individual. In particular, a substantial convection effect is commonly responsible for frostbite of the face, particularly the ears and nose, as well as the fingers.

Respiration has a limited role in thermoregulation. Heat transfer is determined by the amount of heat needed to warm inhaled air in the bronchi and alveoli in the winter or the amount of heat gained from the heated air of summer.

Radiation is determined by the thermal gradient between the environment and the body independent of air currents or direct contact. In summer the short-wave radiant heat received directly from or reflected by the sun is balanced by the long-wave radiation given off by the human body.

Evaporation is generally considered solely a mechanism of heat loss. It is most consequential in the summer, when, as the ambient temperature rises, evaporation becomes the major mechanism of heat loss. The temperature-humidity index (THI) reflects the interactions between temperature and humidity. As this index increases, evaporation decreases and a high risk period for heat stroke prevails. Many of the drugs utilized by homeless patients effect sweating and therefore evaporation. Excretion of urine and feces has little impact on thermal control.

PHARMACOLOGIC AND TOXICOLOGIC INTERACTIONS WITH THERMOREGULATION

The vast majority of patients, and the homeless in particular, are exposed to drugs and toxins, primarily ethanol and nicotine. Diverse drugs of abuse—such as central nervous system stimulants (PCP, amphetamines), opioids (methadone and heroin), and sedative hypnotics—are used by the younger homeless patients.[3] Psychotropic agents frequently prescribed by the providers of health care for the homeless include phenothiazines, butyrophenones, and tricyclic antidepressants. Many of these drugs dramatically alter the individual's ability to perceive and respond appropriately to thermal environmental stress. These pharmacologic alterations affect both the central and peripheral nervous systems and have direct effects on the muscles, sweat glands, and blood vessels as well. (See Table 4.2.)

Ethanol is known by all for its effects on the central nervous system. A logical approach to the environment is difficult in the intoxicated state.[4] Intoxicated people may perceive the effect of effort and the degree of heat inaccurately. The consequence may be a dramatic increase in either heat gain or heat loss, depending on the environmental conditions. In winter the ethanol-induced vasodilatation leads to increased loss of heat to the environment, a response opposite to that desired. In summer excessive vasodilatation may allow for inappropriate absorption of heat from the environment. Abuse of ethanol is invariably associated with serious metabolic abnormalities. Ethanol may be used to replace all other caloric intake, leading to deficits in protein, carbohy-

Table 4.2. Thermoregulatory Interference

Drug	CNS Stimulation	Uncoupled Oxidated Phosp.	Peripheral Vasocon-striction	↑Muscular Heat Production	Decreased Sweating
Amphetamine	X		X	X	
Cocaine	X		X	X	
Salicylates	X	X			
Antihistamines					X
Atropine					X
Phenothiazines				X	
Lithium	X			X	
Phencyclidine	X			X	
EtOH Withdrawal	X			X	
Inhalation anesthesia				X (MH)	
Succinyl choline				X (MH)	
Pancuronium bromide				X (MH)	
Tricyclic antidepressants	X			X	X

(From Goldfrank LR, Flomenbaum N, Lewin N, Weisman RS. Nonseasonal Heatstroke. Hospital Physician. 1982; 18(6): 50–70. Copyright © by PW Communications, 1982. Reprinted with permission.)

drates, fats, vitamins, and minerals. These deficits produce serious injuries to muscles, vessels, and nerves. Hypothermia due to thermoregulatory instability is a typical manifestation of the Wernicke-Korsakoff syndrome and thiamine depletion.[5]

Cigarette smoking and the absorption of nicotine alter the body's response to the environment. Nicotine can lead to severe vasoconstriction and further impair the vascular supply to an extremity already compromised by cold. Restriction of cigarette smoking in patients with cold injury has important clinical implications. The other toxins of abuse—such as barbiturates, methaqualone, ethchlorvynol, heroin, and methadone—have a major effect in decreasing perception of the environment. These toxins usually enhance the risk of exposure to environmental extremes. It must be remembered, however, that withdrawal from these substances places the individual at risk for temperature elevation.

Psychoactive drugs are the most commonly associated with hyperthermia. The major effects may include alteration of the role of the anterior hypothalamus, increased muscular activity, and decreased sweating. The phenothiazines and butyrophenones may result in a poikilothermic state, with environmental changes leading to dramatic temperature shifts. These agents may lead to a decrease in shivering, which may decrease heat production; but excessive muscular activity such as dystonic reactions, the neuroleptic malignant syndrome, and tardive dyskinesias may place these patients at great risk. The anticholinergic effects can lead to a loss of evaporation as a heat dissipating mechanism, a phenomenon which places these patients at an exceedingly high risk in summer.

COLD-RELATED ILLNESSES

Even in the homeless patient, etiologies other than exposure must always be considered in the differential diagnosis of the hypothermic state.[6-8] (See Table 4.3.)

The true incidence of hypothermia is difficult to determine, but 2 to 3 percent of elderly patients are found hypothermic in their homes.[9] The woman in Figure 4.1 is surrounded by her belongings and the critical problems relating to her attempt to achieve thermoregulation. Exposure alone can lead to any of the cold-related disorders, but the impact of the additional factors of pharmacology, toxicology, vasomotor control, neurology, metabolism, psychology, economics, and nutrition makes the risks and complications all the more consequential.

Table 4.3. Risks for Hypothermia

Environmental exposure
    water, wind, temperature
Endocrine disorders
    diabetes (coma, acidosis), Addison's disease, myxedema, hypopituitarism
Dermatologic disorders
    erythroderma
Chronic debilitating diseases
    cirrhosis, starvation, chronic renal failure, congestive heart failure
CNS disorders
    CVA, hypothalamic disorders
Nutritional deficits
    Wernicke-Korsakoff syndrome
Toxins
    ethanol, sedatives, CNS depressants, carbon monoxide
Psychotropic agents
    phenothiazines, tricyclic antidepressants
Trauma
Impaired environmental perception

Hypothermia

A hypothermic state is defined by a core body temperature of less than 35°C (95°F), determined by careful recording of the rectal temperature. All other means of determining temperature (axillary, oral) are notoriously unreliable. Because hypothermic patients may be agitated and confused, a rectal thermocouple probe should be used. This type of measuring device has a range from 60°–115°F, whereas standard hospital glass thermometers not only may have a limited range excluding the extremes of temperature, but also may be fractured if the patient is uncooperative.

The hypothermic patient has diverse manifestations of metabolic failure.[10,11] (See Table 4.4.) Mild hypothermia (35–32.2°C or 95–90°F) is not usually a major risk to the patient. The patient looses coordination, often falls, and has a limited ability to react appropriately. Mentation is not gravely impaired, although dysarthria is a common finding. Shivering is usually present. These patients are often initially presumed to be intoxicated. As the temperature falls further, into a more critical range of 32.2–25.6°C (90–78.2°F), shivering stops and muscular rigidity ensues. Delirium, stupor, or coma commonly occur. Often, life-threatening cardiac dysrhythmias are noted.[12] Severe metabolic impairment, metabolic acidosis, respiratory depression, impaired renal function, pancreatitis, and thrombotic complications are found. Neither the length of time that the patient has been in the hypothermic state nor the extent of hypothermia is considered a prognostic factor, although the longer the patient requires supportive care, the greater the potential for complications. Patients with other serious health problems clearly are at additional risk from hypothermia.[4]

Patient management is usually hospital based, although care can and certainly should start in the field. (See Figure 4.2.) Resuscitation implies basic life support. Cardiopulmonary stability must be established, but we should recognize that profound bradycardia and/or hypotension are potentially appropriate metabolic responses to hypothermia. Patients should be removed immediately from a cold wet environment. Wet garments should be replaced by dry clothes and blankets. Glucose (50 percent dextrose in water) and thiamine are essential therapeutics. Beyond these points, there is extensive debate about treatment, with particular

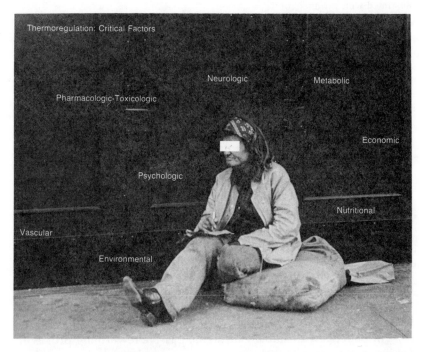

Figure 4.1. A Homeless Woman on the Streets of New York. The critical factors defining thermoregulation are found in the text. (Reprinted with permission of the photographer.)

Table 4.4. Major Symptom Stages and Clinical Manifestations of Hypothermia

MAJOR SYMPTOM STAGES

Mild hypothermia (35 to 32.2 C): Usually a quite benign state: slight clumsiness, slowed response to any stimuli, and dysarthria are common, but the body may compensate adequately. Shivering starts at this stage.

Significant hypothermia (32.2 to 25.6 C): Shivering stops and is replaced by muscular rigidity. Delirium, stupor, and coma may be present.

Severe hypothermia (lower than 25.6 C): Death may ensue if prolonged.

CLINICAL MANIFESTATIONS

Depressed CNS function; depressed metabolism; metabolic acidosis; cardiovascular depression; bradycardia, hypotension, myocardial necrosis, arrhythmias; respiratory depression; decreased renal function; leukocytosis; normal endocrine function (thyroid in particular); pancreatitis; elevated serum muscle enzyme values; thrombotic complication.

(From Goldfrank LR, Kirstein R. Hypothermia. In Goldfrank LR, ed. Toxicologic emergencies: a comprehensive handbook in problem solving, 2nd Edition. New York: Appleton-Century-Crofts, 1982: 194. Copyright © by Appleton-Century-Crofts, 1982. Reprinted with permission.)

dispute about the virtues of active internal as opposed to passive external rewarming.[8] Many authorities choose passive external rewarming when the patient has a stable hemodynamic status; that is, all conditions other than ventricular fibrillation, ventricular tachycardia, or asystole.[13,14] Patients with the latter conditions should be actively rewarmed by any technique available. These may include a warming fan, warming ventilator,[15] warmed nasogastric fluids, warmed IV fluids, warmed rectal fluids, warmed thoracic or peritoneal lavage fluids.[16] Others have utilized a warm Hubbard bath, although this may be a risk with an uncooperative patient. For these critically ill patients we believe that pharmacologic agents have little effect, particularly at very low body temperatures (less than 85°F), and that resuscitation attempts should continue in all patients until the temperature exceeds 95°F. A patient should not be considered dead until he is warm and dead. The resuscitation effort, often lengthy, is usually performed with an oxygen-driven CPR device such as the "Thumper." This facilitates care without immobilizing an entire emergency department or intensive care unit.

For patients with stable vital signs, passive rewarming proves effective. Some workers feel that passive external rewarming may lead to an after-drop in body temperature, with resultant dysrhythmias. We have not found this to be the case when rewarming is performed at a rate of 1 to 2°C/hr. This effort should take place in an intensive care unit, with the patient under close observation for dysrhythmias, infections, and metabolic disorders. Good critical care and supportive efforts allow the survival of 90 to 100 percent of patients with hypothermia due solely to exposure; however, those with any prior serious underlying disorder have a mortality rate of 75 to 90 percent.[4] A major clinical concern in hypothermic patients is the possibility of frostbite or other underlying cutaneous injury. Any damaged areas must be protected as rewarming is instituted.

Frostbite

Frostbite may exist independently of or concomitantly with hypothermia. Exposure to severe cold in the presence of moisture and/or a consequential wind-chill factor dramatically complicates any injury. Environmental exposure is the essential event, although the underlying vasomotor, neurologic, and metabolic characteristics of the extremity (nose, ears, fingers, or toes) play a critical role.[17] Although uncovered and exposed areas are at greatest risk, larger parts of the body can develop frostbite if the period of exposure is extended.

Frostbite may be graded from first to fourth degrees, depending upon whether the epidermis only is involved or a full thickness injury is found.[18,19] First-degree frostbite is the most benign presentation and is manifested by paraesthesias, dysesthesias, and a whitened skin rapidly returning to normal color with a flush upon rewarming. When the

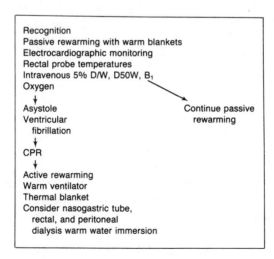

Figure 4.2. Treatment for Hypothermia

frostbite is more substantial, the neurovascular and muscular tissues are impaired and have a doughy consistency. This tissue usually remains viable, and neither bullae nor necrosis ensues. Swelling, hypersensitivity to cold, and erythema are noted for days to weeks.

Second-degree frostbite is marked by bullae that appear hemorrhagic, and necrotic. These areas are easily injured, ultimately leading to infection and long-term tissue loss. Excellent local care is essential to minimize tissue loss. Dysesthesias, paraesthesias, hypersensitivity to cold, edema, and vasodilatation are noted as sequellae.

Third-degree injuries are necrotic in nature. Muscle and connective tissue appear woody and cadaveric. Neurovascular impairment is grave, and only weeks of care and observation determine whether sensation and function will be regained or whether demarcation and auto-amputation will ensue. The cellular consequences of local cooling are limited unless freezing has occurred. Freezing rapidly leads to functional and structural destruction of cells. Extracellular crystals develop, leading to increasing extracellular osmolarity with subsequent osmotic gradients. As intracellular crystallization proceeds, cell destruction with protein denaturation ensues. If rapid tissue thawing is not accomplished prior to this cycle, tissue necrosis will result.

Treatment of frostbite must be rapid and can be initiated in the field by contact rewarming.[19] Only a critical life-threatening condition takes precedence. Rewarming must be done in the field only if there is no risk of refreezing en route to the hospital. Remove the patient from a cold environment, do not give nicotine, and remove constraining garments. Do not rub, thaw in hot water nor rewarm under direct heat. Once in the hospital, rapid rewarming in a large water basin with water at a temperature from 38–42°C (100–110°F) should thaw the extremity rapidly. Local care, restriction of cigarettes, good nutrition and occupational therapy play a critical role in success.[20]

Trench Boot

This entity is one of the commoner environmental disorders found in the homeless. Trench boot has been termed "immersion foot" or "deep-seated cold injury." Known under many other names as well, it is directly related to prolonged exposure to cold and damp, typically in the moist environment of winter boots. The individual may warm a fully covered foot in front of a fire or stove, sweat in dirty socks and shoes (or sneakers)—and the vicious cycle has started. It will be complicated by the effects of snow, rain, and cold. There is neither time, place, nor finances to bathe and dry the feet and to change footwear, essential practices to prevent bacterial growth, cold-induced vasoconstriction, dependency, immobility, and resultant tissue hypoxia leading to ischemia. This process is clearly related to the enhanced heat-conduction ability of water, twenty times greater than that of dry air, which leads to dramatic heat loss. The initial phase of ischemia may not be noted by the patient; or, instead, sensation may be lost early and a cold, waxy, mottled, cyanotic, pulseless extremity may be uncovered on the first assessment. Some patients, when diagnosed at this early stage, develop a hyperemic state weeks later with the development of erythema, edema, pain, and bullae. Those who present later may have gross tissue destruction with myonecrosis leading to risk of tetanus and immediate surgical intervention. Those patients who do recover manifest hyperhydrosis, dysesthesias, excessive sensitivity to cold, and muscular weakness. In this case, proper care entails local hygiene (warming, drying, and washing), protection from tetanus, limitation of weight bearing, analgesics, and antibiotics.[10]

HEAT-RELATED ILLNESSES

There are three major heat-related illnesses.[21,22] (See Table 4.5.) Of these, heat stroke is life-threatening, while heat exhaustion (heat prostration) and heat cramps are debilitating but rarely associated with major complications. Heat stroke is a major risk for the homeless during hot and humid weather[23] or at any time for those homeless who are receiving pharmacologic agents[24] affecting thermoregulation. (See Table 4.2.) Those who are aged,[25,26] homeless, debilitated, and malnourished with underlying chronic diseases are at grave risk when the Temperature-Humidity Index increases.[27] In particular, diseases such as diabetes mellitus, chronic and acute psychiatric disorders, cardiovascular disease, neurologic disorders (Parkinson's disease), and dermatologic disorders place patients at increased risk. (See Table 4.6.) Use of many of the psychotropic agents (lithium, tricyclic antidepressants, phenothiazines) can lead to thermoregulatory disorders.[28-32]

Some of the underlying conditions found in the epidemiologic studies of the heat wave and subsequent heat stroke cases in Saint Louis and Kansas City in 1980 were related to twentieth century adaptive mechanisms that the homeless lack.[33] Most people seek air conditioned, cooled, dehumidified homes, workplaces, stores, and public transportation for some part of their day. Most individuals increase air conditioning in times of thermal stress. The homeless not only lack ac-

Table 4.5. Differential Diagnosis of Heat Syndromes

	Heatstroke (Most severe)	Exhaustion (Prostration—Moderate)	Cramps (Mild)
INDIVIDUALS AFFECTED	Aged, debilitated, or malnourished persons, particularly those with chronic diseases including renal, cerebrovascular, parkinsonism, diabetes, alcoholism, obesity, and dermatologic diseases. Also: drug (particularly amphetamine) abusers, and over-exertion in healthy individuals.	Sedendary, poorly acclimatized individuals, particularly after exercise. Volume-depleted patients or those on diuretic therapy are at especially high risk. Associated with cardio-vascular disease.	Adequately acclimatized young patients in good physical condition. Usually occurs during performance of intense physical activity. Rarely seen in elderly patients.
MECHANISM	Relative or absolute of thermoregulation.	Inadequate autonomic and cardiovascular response to circulatory changes. (a) Water depletion is greater than salt depletion. (b) Salt depletion is greater than water depletion.	Excessive loss of NaCl→skeletal muscle cramps.

SYMPTOMS	Headache, weakness, confusion, delirium, coma, death. Hyperthermia (not necessarily preceded by exhaustion or cramps).	Anorexia, nausea, vomiting, faintness, weakness, occasional cramps, myalgias, postural hypotension: often disoriented. (a) Increased temperature. (b) Normal or slightly decreased temperature.	Mental status normal. Painful muscle contractions. Temperature normal.
SKIN	Elderly: often hot, dry (anhidrotic) Young: frequently hot, moist.	Moist, pale, clammy.	Cool, moist.
THERAPY	Ice bath (see discussion). Admit all patients.	Cool environment, H_2O, NaCl, PO or IV. Rest for 48 hr.	Cool environment, H_2O, NaCL, PO, rest. Observation. Avoid exertion for 24 hr.
MORTALITY	High.	Rare.	None.

(From Goldfrank LR, Osborn H, Weisman R. Heat stroke in toxicologic emergencies: a comprehensive handbook in problem solving. 2nd edition. New York: Appleton-Century-Crofts, 1982: 206. Copyright © by Appleton-Century-Crofts, 1982. Reprinted with permission.)

Table 4.6. Risks for Heat Stroke

Environment exposure
    temperature, humidity
Psychotropic agents
    tricyclic antidepressants, phenothiazines, lithium
Chronic diseases
    CNS, heart, lungs, kidneys, diabetes
Nutritional deficits
Acute and chronic motor disorders
Trauma
Impaired environmental perception
Toxins
Psychiatric disorders
Dermatologic disorders

---

cess to those areas for cooling but have no access to showers or baths. Other major risk factors include the extent of trees or shrubs near patients' living quarters, height above ground level of floor of residence, and adaptive characteristics such as taking of extra fluids, decreasing activity levels, and being able to render self-care. Both intoxication and withdrawal from alcohol, and the associated agitation, commonly lead to heat-stroke-like states. The use of psychotropic agents is one of the more prevalent complicating factors.[34] This is often difficult to dissociate epidemiologically from the underlying psychiatric disorder.

Heat stroke develops because of thermoregulatory failure.[21,22,35-37] Heat stroke is defined by a temperature greater than 105°F (40.6°C), neurologic impairment (delirium, stupor, or coma), and a hot dry skin. Patients typically have few premonitory signs. A headache, weakness, and altered consciousness may precede the fully blown syndrome. Rarely, heat exhaustion or heat cramps precede heat stroke. Management is defined quite simply by Figure 4.3 and Table 4.5. The elevation of temperature beyond a specific level, such as 105°F, must be considered a life-threatening emergency necessitating immediate intervention. Although one may simultaneously consider infectious etiologies, the patient's temperature must be lowered immediately with an ice bath.[38] Many techniques have been suggested for lowering the core temperature, such as body lavage with water or alcohol, nasogastric lavage with cool fluids, cooled IV fluids, dialysis, and cooling blankets.[21,22] None of these cover the total body surface area as effectively as does an ice bath. Pharmacologic agents should not be used in the management, as they may further complicate the critical care setting, may not be metabolized, and have not been proven beneficial. An ice bath can rapidly return a patient to a normal mental status. A temperature as high as 110–112°F can be returned to a temperature of 101–102°F within twenty to forty minutes. This rapid response is necessary to preserve compromised tissue,[39] particularly brain, liver, skeletal muscle, and myocardium.[40,41]

Hepatic necrosis, rabdomyolysis,[42] and cellular destruction in the central nervous system are noted in the heat stroke state. Supportive care is essential if these patients are to survive, but rapid intervention can lead to an 85 percent survival rate with limited morbidity.

Heat exhaustion is a common summer syndrome among those patients with intercurrent disease leading to volume depletion, such as gastroenteritis or alcohol withdrawal. In those patients with chronic renal failure or chronic congestive heart failure[26] who do not alter their fluid intake in spite of increasing sodium and water losses due to sweating, heat exhaustion is common. These individuals have moist, clammy

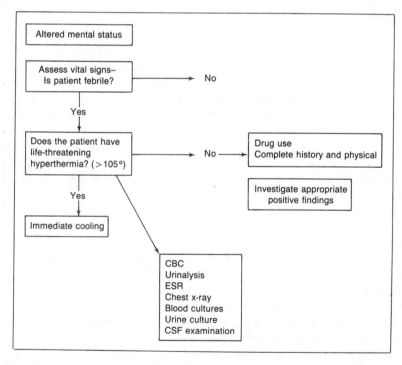

Figure 4.3. Managing Heat-Related Illness (From Goldfrank LR, Flomenbaum N, Lewin N, Weisman RS. Nonseasonal heatstroke. Hospital Physician. 1982; 18(6):50–70. Copyright © by PW Communications, 1982. Reprinted with permission.)

skin, anorexia, nausea, vomiting, faintness, cramps, myalgias, mild temperature elevation (101–102°F), and orthostatic hypotension.[43,44]

For treatment, sodium chloride and water repletion are needed, as well as rest. Mortality is rare. After volume depletion, central nervous system and cardiovascular compromise is the major concern.

Heat cramps may occur in older patients who overextend themselves in the face of the extremes of heat and humidity.[45] Excessive loss of sodium chloride and water leads to rapid extracellular osmolar shifts, which in turn leads to muscular cramps. These can be painful but are usually rapidly corrected by a cool environment, water repletion, and sodium chloride repletion. Rest and observation prove quite adequate and hospitalization is unnecessary. Mortality is not noted and morbidity is limited.

PREVENTION OF HEAT-RELATED ILLNESSES

In considering the homeless, health providers must evaluate their patients' impaired psychological, nutritional, dermatologic, neurologic, vasomotor, and metabolic states. These factors, when abnormal, deny patients the opportunity for appropriate adjustment to thermal stresses.

The following are general guidelines to prevention of heat- and cold-related illnesses:[39]

1. Prepare for environmental stress by making air conditioners and baths available in shelters each summer. Make sure shelters are warm and dry when the weather is cold and wet.

2. Change the level of activity during extremely warm or cold periods. Decrease activity when heat stroke and hypothermia are great risks.

3. Change the type and amount of clothing and bedding on a seasonal basis. Remove dangerous clothing such as plastics in summer, emphasizing airy and cool clothing. Provide arctic attire for the winter. Change shoes and socks frequently.

4. Consider the appropriate level of high-risk medications. Doses of antipsychotic drugs, antidepressants, and diuretics for congestive heart failure must vary depending on the season.

5. Have a health care team available to plan management and care, with particular emphasis on environmental stress. Education with regard to the aforementioned issues is essential. This might be called a code of daily living in the face of environmental flux.

6. If homeless activities are organized, plan them for the coolest and least humid time of the day in summer. The pace of work must be adjusted to the capacity of the individual to acclimatize.[22,46]

7. Be particularly careful for those patients with intellectual and psychiatric impairment, those with trouble in previous years in adapting to the environment, those who are overweight and those with drug utilization of any sort and in particular those who are alcoholic.

A concerted effort to prepare for environmental variations is necessary to prevent the homeless from suffering from what often becomes an irreversible, yet preventable, medical catastrophe.

REFERENCES

1. Goldfrank LR, Kirstein R. Hypothermia. Toxicologic emergencies: a comprehensive handbook to problem solving. New York: Appleton-Century-Crofts, 1982:189–99.
2. MacLean D, Emslie-Smith D. Accidental hypothermia. London: Blackwell, 1977.
3. Fell RH, Gunning AJ, Bardhan KD, Triger DR. Severe hypothermia as a result of barbiturate overdose complicated by cardiac arrest. Lancet. 1968; 1:392–94.
4. Weyman AE, Greenbaum DM, Grace WJ. Accidental hypothermia in an alcoholic population. Am J Med. 1974; 56:13–20.
5. Koeppen AH, Daniels JC, Barron KD. Subnormal body temperatures in Wernicke's encephalopathy. Neurology. 1969; 21:493–98.
6. Fruehan AE. Accidental hypothermia. Arch Intern Med. 1960; 106: 218–29.
7. Hudson LD, Conn RD. Accidental hypothermia: associated diagnoses and prognosis in a common problem. JAMA. 1974; 227:37–40.
8. O'Keefe KM. Accidental hypothermia: a review of 62 cases. JACEP. 1977; 6:491–96.
9. Fox RH, Woodward PM, Exton-Smith AN. Body temperature in the elderly: a national study of physiological, social and environmental conditions. Brit Med J. 1973; 1:200–206.
10. Pozos RS, Wittmers LE, eds. The nature and treatment of hypothermia. Vol. 2. Minneapolis: University of Minnesota Press, 1983.
11. Reuler JB. Hypothermia: Pathophysiology, clinical settings and management. Ann Intern Med. 1978; 89:519–27.
12. Trevino A, Razi B, Beller BM. The characteristic electrocardiogram of accidental hypothermia. Arch Intern Med. 1971; 127:470–73.
13. Collis ML, Steinman AM, Chaney RD. Accidental hypothermia: an experimental study of practical rewarming methods. Aviat Space Environment Med. 1977; 48:625–32.

14. Miller JW, Danzl DF, Thomas DM. Urban accidental hypothermia: 135 cases. Ann Emerg Med. 1980; 9:456–61.
15. Hayward JS, Steinman AM. Accidental hypothermia: an experimental study of inhalation rewarming. Aviat Space Environ Med. 1975; 46:1236–40.
16. Jessen K, Hagelston JO. Peritoneal dialysis in the treatment of profound accidental hypothermia. Aviat Space Environ Med. 1978; 49:426–29.
17. Bangs CC, Boswick JA, Hamlet MP, Sumner DS, Weatherly-White RCA. When your patient suffers frostbite. Patient Care. 1977; 11:132–56.
18. Killian H. Cold and frost injuries: rewarming damages biological, angiological, and clinical aspects. In: Frey R, Safar P, eds. Disaster medicine, vol. 3. New York: Springer-Verlag, 1981.
19. Lapp NL, Juergens JL. Frostbite. Mayo Clin Proc. 1965; 40:932–38.
20. Mills WJ Jr. Frostbite. Alaska Med. 1973; 15(2):27–47.
21. Goldfrank LR, Osborn H, Weisman RS. Heat stroke in toxicologic emergencies: a comprehensive handbook in problem solving. New York: Appleton-Century-Crofts, 1982:201–11.
22. Knochel JP. Environmental heat illness: an eclectic review. Arch Intern Med. 1974; 133:841–64.
23. Bridges CA, Ellis FP, Taylor HL. Mortality in St. Louis Missouri during heat waves in 1936, 1953, 1954, 1955 and 1956-Coroner Case. Environ Res. 1976; 12:38–48.
24. McAllister RG. Fever, tachycardia and hypertension with acute catatonic schizophrenia. Arch Intern Med. 1978; 138:1154–56.
25. Levine JA. Heat stroke in the aged. Am J Med. 1968; 47:251–58.
26. Strung CL. Hemodynamic alterations of heat stroke in the elderly. Chest. 1979; 75:362–66.
27. Bacon C, Scott D, Jones P. Heat stroke in well-wrapped infants. Lancet. 1979; 1:422–25.
28. Granoff AL, Davis JM. Heat illness syndrome and lithium intoxication. J Clin Psychol. 1978; 39:103–107.
29. Ginsberg MD, Hertzman M, Schmidt-Nowara WW. Amphetamine intoxication with coagulopathy, hyperthermia and reversible renal failure: a syndrome resembling heat stroke. Ann Intern Med. 1970; 73:81–85.
30. Krisko I et al. Severe hyperpyrexia due to tranylcypromine-amphetamine toxicity. Ann Intern Med. 1969; 70:559–63.
31. Maickel RP. Interaction of drugs with autonomic nervous function and thermoregulation. Fed Proc. 1970; 29:1973–79.
32. Greenland P, Southwick WH. Hyperthermia associated with chlorpromazine and full sheet restraint. Am J Psychiatry. 1978; 135:1234–35.
33. Jones TS, Liang AP, Kilbourne EM, et al. Morbidity and mortality associated with July 1980 heat wave in St. Louis and Kansas City Missouri. JAMA. 1982; 247:3327–31.
34. Goldfrank LR, Flomenbaum N, Lewin N, Weisman RS. Nonseasonal heatstroke. Hospital Physician. 1982; 18(6):50–70.
35. Clowes GHA, O'Donnell TF. Heat stroke. N Engl J Med. 1974; 291:565–66.
36. Gottschalk PG, Thomas JE. Heat stroke. Mayo Clin Proc. 1966; 41:470–82.

37. Eichler AC, McFee AS, Root HD. Heat stroke. Am J Surg. 1969; 118:855–63.
38. Berheim HA et al. Fever: pathogenesis, pathophysiology and purpose. Ann Intern Med. 1979; 91:261–70.
39. Knochel JP, Caskey JH. The mechanism of hypophosphatemia in acute heat stroke. JAMA. 1977; 238:425–26.
40. Costrini AM, Pitt MA, Gustafson AB. Cardiovascular and metabolic manifestations of heat stroke and severe heat exhaustion. Am J Med. 1979; 66: 296–302.
41. O'Donnel TJ, Clowes GHA. The circulatory abnormalities of heat stroke. N Engl J Med. 1972; 287:734–37.
42. Knochel JP, Dotin LN, Hamburger RJ. Heat stress exercise and muscle injury: effects on urate metabolism and renal function. Ann Intern Med. 1974; 81:321–28.
43. Shibolet S, Coll R, Gilat T, Sohar E. Heat stroke: its clinical picture and mechanism in 36 cases. Q J Med. 1967; 36:525–48.
44. Shibolet S, Lancaster MC, Danon Y. Heat stroke: a review. Aviat Space Environ Med. 1976; 47:280–301.
45. Wheeler M. Heat stroke in the elderly. Med Clin North Am. 1976; 60: 1289–96.
46. Shapiro Y, Magazanik H, Udassin R. Heat intolerance in former heat stroke patients. Ann Intern Med. 1979; 90:913–16.

5

Trauma: With the Example of San Francisco's Shelter Programs

John T. Kelly

Trauma is one of the leading causes of death and disability among the homeless. Without safe refuge, and with faculties impaired by alcohol and mental illness, the homeless are vulnerable and particularly susceptible to injuries. Once injured, they may lack access to adequate medical services. Their recovery may be hampered by malnutrition, exposure, or inadequate follow-up care.

There are few analyses of the kinds of injuries the homeless suffer. A Stockholm study of mortality among 6032 homeless men found that of 327 deaths during a three-year period, almost 20 percent were a result of trauma (falls, accidents, poisoning, drowning, or murder), a cause of death twelve times that expected for age-matched controls.[1] A study of 227 homeless, chronic alcoholics in Toronto revealed a remarkably high incidence of fractures: 30.4 percent had previous limb fractures, 18.9 percent had previous rib fractures, and 14.1 percent had previous skull fractures.[2]

Other indigent people, such as single-room-occupancy (SRO) hotel residents, many of whom are intermittently homeless, are also at great risk of trauma.[3] In a clinic in a large welfare hotel in New York City, trauma was the presenting complaint of almost 20 percent of the patients. Of the injuries treated, accidents accounted for 52 percent, assaults accounted for 41 percent, and burns accounted for the remainder.[4]

The treatment of trauma among the homeless is complex and multifaceted. Prehospital care, emergency services, inpatient care, and outpatient follow-up are each important components of an effective trauma management system.

TREATING MAJOR TRAUMA

In all major trauma, definitive treatment must be initiated within minutes to be successful. The gravity of the problem must be identified by the victim or those with him. Emergency help must be sought, usually by calling for an ambulance. Ambulance dispatchers and drivers must understand the severity of the situation and respond rapidly. Paramedics must correctly identify the severity of the victim's condition, initiate life-saving measures, and quickly transport the victim to an appropriate facility.

In dramatic injuries to the homeless, such as stabbings or shootings, this complex sequence of interventions often occurs successfully. However, the homeless are also victims of less dramatic but nonetheless major injuries, such as closed head trauma. Observers might incorrectly assume that an unconscious transient on a curb or at the bottom of a flight of stairs is intoxicated when he may in fact have sustained major injuries. Even if injuries are recognized, the homeless often lack ready access to telephones to summon immediate help. Ambulance dispatchers, often inundated with calls from skid row, may fail to send an ambulance promptly. Paramedics at the scene might attribute a homeless victim's condition to alcohol or drugs rather than to injuries. Other homeless trauma victims, such as those who are loners or who live in deserted buildings, might not be discovered until long after they have sustained injuries.

When a homeless trauma victim arrives in the emergency department, the initial treatment should be identical to that for any other patient: evaluation of respiratory and circulatory status; acquisition of a relevant history; performance of a thorough physical examination, including careful evaluation of mental status; identification of all injuries, and appropriate treatment. For major trauma, this includes the introduction of life-saving measures such as endotracheal intubation and fluid resuscitation.[5]

Full patient evaluation is a fundamental principle that cannot be violated. Victims must be recognized as homeless. All injuries and complicating conditions common among the homeless, such as hypothermia or metabolic disorders, must be recognized. Of special concern are alterations in states of consciousness, which are exceedingly common among patients who are alcoholics or drug abusers, are mentally disturbed, or have suffered head injuries; all are possibilities that must be carefully considered. Patients who are infested, disorderly, paranoid, or uncooperative must likewise be fully evaluated, even if treating such patients may be difficult or unpleasant.

After initial treatment, all major trauma victims, especially those with severe multisystem injuries, prolonged hypotension, or preexisting cardiovascular or respiratory disease, remain at considerable risk. Postoperative complications are common and include hemorrhage, shock, sepsis, respiratory failure, pulmonary embolism, renal failure, myocardial infarction, and death.[6,7]

While it is appropriate in the early management of major trauma to focus on treatable acute problems, it is essential in the recovery phase to consider how conditions such as homelessness itself, alcoholism, drug abuse, and mental illness might interfere with recovery or necessitate changes in treatment plans. Does the patient's homelessness necessitate admission even though his injury could be treated in an outpatient facility? Does the patient have medical conditions such as cirrhosis or tuberculosis that might complicate treatment or recovery? Does the patient require a longer than usual hospitalization because he is homeless? Does the patient insist on leaving the hospital before appropriate treatment is completed? Many complicated management issues must be addressed.

TREATING MINOR TRAUMA

Minor trauma is usually not life-threatening. Nevertheless, significant suffering and even permanent disability can occur if minor trauma is not treated appropriately. A victim needs to recognize that he is injured, understand that medical care is required, know where to get treatment, and present at an appropriate facility in order for treatment to be successful.

Homeless persons who are intoxicated or mentally ill may not recognize that they are injured or present for care in a timely manner. Transients may not know where to receive medical help.

Once victims of minor trauma seek medical care, they must be willing to wait until they have been evaluated and treated. Minor trauma is often accorded low priority in busy emergency departments, and many of the homeless leave before treatment is provided. Others do not even seek treatment because they are aware of the long waiting times.

Wound care is of paramount concern among homeless trauma victims because of the high incidence of stab wounds, lacerations, bites, and burns. General principles of initial wound care include removal of dirty clothing; thorough assessment of the type of injury, extent of tissue damage, and presence of foreign bodies or other contamination; careful preparation of the wound, including mechanical cleansing and debridement of contaminated or devitalized tissue; proper closure of the wound; protection of the wound with sterile dressings or splints; and instruction to the patient on wound care and the signs of infection.[5] It is important to assess the patient's general condition because of its impact on healing.

Prophylactic antibiotic therapy as an adjunct to wound care merits special consideration. Prophylaxis is clearly indicated when treatment has been delayed and for wounds, such as bites, that are highly susceptible to infection. Antibiotics are also indicated in patients with debilitating conditions such as diabetes mellitus. Patients who are alcoholic or severely malnourished may also benefit from prophylactic antibiotics. However, homeless patients often fail to fill prescriptions, frequently lose their medications, and regularly neglect to take them. It is preferable to provide medications directly to patients rather than to expect them to have prescriptions filled. Many patients lack the money to purchase even inexpensive medications. It is essential to inform patients of the value of prophylactic drugs and the potential risks if they fail to take such medication. It may be valuable to have patients return daily in order to monitor antibiotic use as well as to check wounds and change dressings.

Tetanus prophylaxis is an important aspect of wound care. The principles of tetanus prophylaxis and the indications for use of tetanus toxoid and human tetanus immune globulin are well established. Among homeless trauma victims, immunization records are generally unavailable and histories of immunization status are often unreliable. Careful consideration should be given to the use of tetanus toxoid. In patients with tetanus-prone wounds, such as contaminated lacerations, special consideration should be given to the use of human tetanus immune globulin.

The management of homeless victims of sexual assault is a complex process that involves evaluation and treatment of physical injuries, assessment of risk of venereal disease and pregnancy, evaluation of psychological response, and collection of legal evidence. It is preferable to provide prophylaxis against venereal disease and unwanted pregnancy on the initial visit rather than to wait for the return of test results; homeless victims of sexual assault rarely return for follow-up and may be impossible to contact. With diligence, the social workers at San Francisco's Sexual Trauma Services (STS) were able to contact more than half of the homeless victims; but less than 9 percent returned to STS for follow-up. It is essential that a victim's homelessness be identified and safe shelter arranged so that the victim is not forced to return to the place in which the assault occurred.

FOLLOW-UP CARE

Follow-up care for homeless trauma victims is especially important. Their circumstances place them at great risk for complications, such as wound infections and delayed healing. Patients who sleep outdoors and lack shower facilities and changes of clothing are rarely able to keep their wounds and dressings clean or their casts intact. Standard practices, such as weekly wound checks or biweekly cast checks, must be altered for the homeless. Ideally, wounds should be checked and dressings changed daily or every other day. Casts should be evaluated frequently.

The homeless generally present infrequently for follow-up care, if at all. Hospital clinics, with limited hours and tight appointment schedules that are often overbooked, are often not well suited to accommodate the lifestyles of the homeless. Emergency departments generally give low priority to follow-up care and often require nonacute patients to wait hours.

Statistics from San Francisco's Central Emergency are typical. Only 21.4 percent of the homeless patients with lacerations that were not infected at the time of initial presentation returned for follow-up wound care. Of the patients with infected lacerations, only 28.6 percent returned for follow-up. As a result, complications, such as chronic infections and prolonged disabilities that often necessitate lengthy hospitalizations, are commonplace.

In planning follow-up care, the single most important need is to identify that patients are homeless, for without such identification effective treatment plans may not be made. When appropriate, homeless patients should be placed in shelters. Other arrangements that can facilitate care include thorough instructions by sympathetic staff that stress the importance of follow-up care; instruction sheets that detail plans for medical care; copies of emergency department records or discharge plans (especially valuable for patients likely to receive follow-up care elsewhere); packets of medications; daily or twice daily dressing changes; regular visits to shelters by professional staff; referrals to facilities with drop-in capability, extended hours, and locations near areas where patients live. Clinics located in the shelters or at the site of meal programs for the homeless are often well adapted for providing care. The employees of shelters, food programs, detoxification centers, social service agencies, and other programs for the homeless are often invaluable to successful follow-up treatment. If the managers and staff of these programs are instructed about the availability of medical services for the homeless, the signs and symptoms of posttraumatic complications, and the indications for referral, they can refer patients who might otherwise not obtain treatment.

The attitudes of the staff are an important factor in providing proper trauma care to the homeless, especially for follow-up treatment. Staff sympathetic to the problems of the homeless, tolerant of their alcohol abuse and mental illness, willing to treat patients who are dirty or infested, and tolerant of their failure to keep appointments are more likely to be influential in encouraging patients to return for medical care. Staff willing to tailor treatment to the needs of the patient are also likely to succeed in encouraging patients to return. If a patient with an infected wound or cellulitis refuses to be hospitalized, it is preferable to treat him as an outpatient rather than to deny treatment altogether.

TREATING SAN FRANCISCO'S HOMELESS

San Francisco's homeless trauma victims receive treatment from a system that is largely defined by the city's institutions, geography, and population. The fourteenth largest city in the United States, San Francisco has a population of 705,408 and occupies 46.4 square miles, a relatively small area. There is one regional trauma center, a single publicly operated, free-standing emergency center, one facility for treating victims of sexual assault, and a coordinated shelter system for the homeless.

According to the 1980 United States Census, 13.7 percent of the population of San Francisco lives below the poverty line. During 1983, over 96,000 individuals in San Francisco received General Assistance (Welfare). More than 10,000 individuals were homeless at some time during 1983, and at least 2000 to 2500 people were homeless on any given day that year, based on the number of clients who utilize the city's emergency shelters and estimates of those who have opted not to use the shelters.

Surveys are conducted monthly of the entire shelter population. Seventy-eight percent are male. Ages range from 18 to 80, with a median of 31.4 years. Fifty-two percent are white, 28 percent black, 11 percent Hispanic, 3 percent American Indian, and 2 percent Asian. Thirty-three percent have been in San Francisco for less than three months, 11 percent from four to six months, 6 percent from seven to eleven months, 10 percent from twelve to twenty-four months, and 38 percent more than two years. Of those who have lived in San Francisco less than twelve months, 42 percent were from California, 37 percent from western and midwestern states, 18 percent from eastern states, and 4 percent from the South. Sixty-nine percent are single, 18 percent divorced or separated, 7 percent married, and 4 percent widowed. These statistics indicate that the homeless population in San Francisco is similar to those in other cities, such as New York, Philadelphia, Washington, and Los Angeles: largely male, single, and transient.[8-14]

Prevalence of Trauma and Trauma-Related Problems

The homeless in San Francisco's emergency shelters have a high incidence of alcohol and drug abuse, mental illness, and disability. In interviews of 170 shelter residents conducted in March 1984, 57.6 percent reported a history of alcohol or drug abuse and 34.7 percent reported previous psychiatric hospitalization. In questionnaires completed by over 200 shelter residents in March 1984, 29 percent reported that they were disabled, with the majority permanently disabled.

City policy requires that all major trauma victims receive treatment at San Francisco General, a 600-bed acute care hospital, which is the regional trauma center. Minor trauma victims who are indigent receive services at San Francisco General Hospital or at Central Emergency, a free-standing facility operated by the San Francisco Department of Public Health and located near the Tenderloin area, where most of the homeless live.[15]

To identify the types of trauma to which the homeless are subjected, the medical records of all patients admitted to San Francisco General Hospital from January 1, 1983, to March 31, 1983, were reviewed. Patients who gave as an address "streets," "transient," or "no local address" were considered homeless and formed the basis of this study. This method, however, excludes patients who were, in fact, homeless but who gave addresses of shelters, former residences, or mailing addresses. Three hundred and forty (7.7 percent) of the 4436 patients admitted during this period were identified as homeless. Of these, fifty-two (15.3 percent) were major trauma victims. Thirty-four other homeless patients (10 percent) were admitted because of cellulitis, often consequent to trauma. Thus, trauma and trauma-related problems accounted for approximately one-quarter of all admissions of homeless patients to San Francisco General Hospital.

The homeless suffer an alarmingly high incidence of repeat trauma and hospitalization. During the three-month period studied, 47 percent of the homeless admitted for major trauma had prior or subsequent hospitalizations at San Francisco General Hospital. Of these patients, over half had been hospitalized for another episode of major trauma. Six percent of the homeless major trauma victims admitted during the three-month period studied were readmitted for a second episode during the same period.

The records of all patients at Central Emergency from January 1, 1983, to June 30, 1983, were reviewed to identify the homeless, using the same criteria as in the San Francisco General Hospital study. Of the 524 homeless patients treated during this period, 156 (30 percent) presented because of trauma, mostly minor.

Trauma victims included homeless men and women of all ages, but were typically males from twenty to thirty-nine years of age. (See Tables 5.1 and 5.2.) They suffered a great variety of severe injuries, including stab wounds, head trauma, blunt trauma, multisystem trauma, gunshots, suicide attempts, burns, complex facial fractures, hip fractures, pneumothoraces, and lacerations of the neck, chest, liver, large and small bowel, and tendons of the hands. Stab wounds and fractures predominated and accounted for 65 percent of the major trauma injuries. (See Table 5.3.)

Many of the homeless major trauma victims had extended hospitalizations and suffered lengthy disabilities. Often their marginal living conditions were directly responsible for complications. A thirty-three-year-old male stabbed in the abdomen had a hospital course complicated by a bowel obstruction that necessitated additional surgery. After his discharge, he returned to the streets and his incision became infected and a dehiscence ensued. As a result, he required subsequent hospitalization. Another homeless victim, a chronic alcoholic who had

Table 5.1. San Francisco General Hospital: Homeless Patients Admitted for Major Trauma (1/1/83–3/31/83)

Age	Male (N = 42)		Female (N = 7)	
20–29	11	26.2%	1	14.3%
30–39	18	42.9%	4	57.1%
40–49	7	16.7%	0	
50–59	3	7.1%	1	14.3%
60 and older	3	7.1%	1	14.3%

Table 5.2. Central Emergency: Homeless Minor Trauma Victims (1/1/83–6/30/83)

Age	Male (N = 138)		Female (N = 18)	
younger than 20	2	1.5%	0	
20–29	37	26.8%	6	33.3%
30–39	64	46.4%	5	27.8%
40–49	17	12.3%	0	
50–59	14	10.1%	3	16.7%
60 and older	4	2.9%	2	11.1%
Unknown			2	11.1%

Table 5.3. San Francisco General Hospital: Homeless Patients Admitted for Major Trauma (1/1/83–3/31/83)*

Primary Reason for Admission	(N = 52)	
Stab wound	19	36.5%
Fracture/dislocation	15	28.8%
Blunt trauma	6	11.5%
Head trauma	5	9.6%
Multisystem trauma	2	3.8%
Gunshot	1	1.9%
Suicide attempt	1	1.9%
Burn	1	1.9%
Bite	1	1.9%
Cellulitis	1	1.9%

*Percentages do not total 100 due to rounding.

a skull fracture, developed chronic cerebrospinal fluid otorrhea and had recurrent bouts of meningitis.

Others developed permanent and severely crippling disabilities. A thirty-three-year-old homeless male became paraplegic from a burst fracture of the first lumbar vertebra sustained when a wall fell on him at a construction site where he slept. A forty-five-year-old homeless victim of head trauma developed a permanent hemiparesis.

The homeless also suffered a great variety of less severe injuries that included bruises; bites; minor burns; sprains; posttraumatic complications such as wound infections; lacerations of the scalp, face, lips, arms, wrists, legs, and feet; and simple fractures of the nose, arms, and legs. Wounds predominated and accounted for 61.6 percent of the injuries attributable to minor trauma. (See Table 5.4.)

Many of the homeless minor trauma victims were injured during assaults. A forty-four-year-old male alcoholic sustained multiple deep facial lacerations during an altercation in which he was attacked with a broken bottle. Some injuries are self-inflicted. A thirty-three-year-old homeless male slashed his wrists during a suicide attempt; several weeks later he lacerated his wrists again in another suicide gesture.

The most frequent complication of these injuries was infection. At Central Emergency, chart review showed that 85 percent of the homeless patients with lacerations for whom the interval from time of injury to time of presentation was documented presented within six hours of

Table 5.4. Central Emergency: Homeless Minor Trauma Victims (1/1/83–6/30/83)*

Reason for Initial Presentation	(N = 172)	
Laceration	70	40.7%
Bruise/contusion	29	16.9%
Post-traumatic cellulitis	19	11.1%
Abrasion	10	5.8%
Bite	8	4.7%
Wound follow-up	7	4.1%
Burn	6	3.5%
Fracture	5	3.5%
Sprain	5	2.9%
Puncture wound	3	1.7%
Suture removal	2	1.2%
Ingestion	2	1.2%
Concussion	2	1.2%
Eye injury	2	1.2%
Arthritis/bursitis	2	1.2%

*Percentages do not total 100 due to rounding.

injury. As a result, lacerations could be cleaned and sutured and the risks of infection reduced. Of the 15 percent who waited more than six hours to present, two-thirds presented more than twenty-four hours after injury and had signs of infection.

The impact of trauma on the homeless is better illustrated by specific examples. A forty-six-year-old homeless male diabetic suffered multiple rib fractures when a garbage truck emptied into its compactor the dumpster in which he was asleep. A thirty-five-year-old homeless female alcoholic sustained a skull fracture when she was beaten and raped by four men in a deserted building where she was sleeping.

The homeless are especially vulnerable to sexual assault. To identify the incidence of sexual assault among the homeless, the records of all patients treated at the Sexual Trauma Service from January 1, 1983, through September 30, 1983, were reviewed. The criteria used to identify which sexual assault victims were homeless were the same as those used in the San Francisco General Hospital and Central Emergency studies. STS, located at Central Emergency and operated by the San Francisco Department of Public Health, is the facility where all adult victims of sexual assault are treated in San Francisco.

Thirty-four patients, over 9 percent of the sexual assault victims treated at STS during the nine-month period studied, were homeless. As the homeless comprise less than 0.4 percent of the population of San Francisco, the incidence of treated sexual assault among the homeless is more than twenty times greater than that of the rest of the population.

Although women make up only 22 percent of the homeless population, they accounted for more than 76 percent of the homeless victims of sexual assault. Most of the victims ranged from twenty to thirty-nine years of age and were subject to a wide range of assaults: 29 percent were vaginal, 15 percent rectal, 3 percent oral, and 41 percent multiple-orifice. (See Table 5.5.) Twelve percent of the assaults were attempts. Half of the victims had injuries, ranging from minor trauma such as sprains and abrasions to major trauma such as skull fractures. All of the victims experienced some degree of psychological trauma.

At STS, 84 percent of the homeless victims of sexual assault for whom the interval between time of assault and time they sought treatment is known presented within twenty-four hours. Consequently, injuries could be evaluated promptly, prophylaxis provided against venereal disease and unwanted pregnancy, and safe shelter arranged.

The incidence of repeat sexual assault among the homeless is also alarming. Twelve percent of the homeless victims of sexual assault

Table 5.5. Sexual Trauma Service: Homeless Victims of Sexual Assault (1/1/83–9/30/83)

Age	Female (N=26)		Male (N=8)	
younger than 20	4	15.4%	2	25.0%
20–29	12	46.2%	5	62.5%
30–39	9	34.6%	1	12.5%
40 and older	1	3.8%	0	

studied had been treated previously at STS for one or more prior sexual assaults.

Medical and Support Systems

The medical system that provides trauma care in San Francisco is complex and presents many obstacles to the homeless. San Francisco General Hospital is located approximately two miles from the downtown area where the food and shelter programs operate and where the homeless spend most of their time. Major trauma victims are usually transported by ambulance, making this geographic separation of relatively little consequence; but minor trauma victims must walk or have the money to pay for bus transportation in order to receive care at San Francisco General. Whereas major trauma victims are treated immediately, minor trauma victims must often wait up to eight hours for treatment in the Emergency Department.

Once patients are discharged from the hospital or the Emergency Department, follow-up care is problematic. Clinic appointments at San Francisco General Hospital are severely limited because of space and fiscal constraints. Waits of several weeks or more are common for appointments to surgery and orthopedic clinics. The outpatient clinics are located at the hospital, which is inconvenient for most of the homeless. Transportation to clinic appointments is unavailable. An impoverished patient must choose between keeping a clinic appointment and eating that day, because there are no food programs near the hospital. Patients who present to the Emergency Department for follow-up care often wait many hours to have a wound checked or a dressing changed.

Central Emergency is more accessible to patients, because it is located near the area where they live. Treatment is available around-the-clock without an appointment. Waiting time is usually less than fifteen minutes. Central Emergency is excellent for wound checks and dressing changes. However, the staff at Central Emergency do not have access to patient records at San Francisco General Hospital, nor is there radiographic or laboratory capability.

A complex variety of support programs plays an important role in the delivery of services to the homeless in San Francisco. The Emergency Shelter System, established in 1982, is the keystone program. Supervised cooperatively by the Mayor's Office and the Department of Social Services, the Emergency Shelter System allocates approximately 400 cots at the Salvation Army, Saint Vincent de Paul Society, Hospitality House, and the Episcopal Sanctuary, as well as 800 beds in residential hotels. Additional hotel beds are rented when demand increases, so that everyone who requests shelter from the Emergency Shelter System is served. The hotel rooms are given preferentially to people with serious medical conditions and to families with children. Recuperating homeless trauma victims, including those discharged from San Francisco General Hospital and those treated as outpatients at San Francisco General Hospital, Central Emergency, and STS, are provided with clean and safe quarters. Shower and bathroom facilities are especially helpful for victims with wounds.

The shelter staffs play important supporting roles in the delivery of medical services. Staff members, often formerly homeless themselves, have been taught by San Francisco Department of Health representatives to summon emergency aid, to care for a patient until an ambulance arrives, and to recognize minor trauma as well as other emergencies that may not be life-threatening but require medical care. The shelters have medical supplies, including basins, wound-cleaning solutions, antibiotic ointments, and dressings, with which the shelter staffs can administer first aid and assist shelter residents in providing follow-up wound care.

Student nurses assist each of the shelter staffs several nights each week. They provide first aid and follow-up care, help patients and staff identify the required treatment, and refer patients to appropriate facilities, usually at San Francisco General Hospital or Central Emergency.

This comprehensive program of support services for the homeless greatly facilitates the recuperation of trauma victims. In addition, because of close cooperation between the shelters and representatives of the San Francisco Department of Public Health, the medical needs of the homeless, as individuals and as a group, are reviewed on an ongoing basis. Because of the strong commitment of the San Francisco Department of Public Health, the range of medical services available to the homeless is continually being improved.

The shelter program has been cost-effective as well as humanitarian. The cost of providing a hotel or shelter to 100 people nightly is less than trauma care for one patient for one day at San Francisco General Hospital. Because of the availability of safe facilities in which patients can recuperate, trauma victims can be discharged earlier from San Francisco General Hospital. Patients recovering in the shelters develop fewer complications, such as wound infections and cellulitis, than do patients discharged to the streets. Patients who do develop complications are usually referred for and receive care earlier than those who live on the streets.

TRAUMA AMONG THE HOMELESS

The homeless are multiply disadvantaged. They lack shelter, food, clothing, and social supports, and they are at great risk for trauma. Once injured, they face enormous obstacles to recovery. Unless medical care is available at facilities accessible to them, with drop-in capabilities and sympathetic staff, homeless trauma victims may not receive essential treatment, may develop preventable complications, and their condition may further deteriorate.

Many homeless do not seek medical care until they have been injured. However, others obtain treatment for a wide range of problems unrelated to trauma, such as infestations and upper respiratory infections. Often the patient's homelessness is not identified and, more often, no effort is made to address the patient's homelessness as a problem. Physicians, nurses, and support personnel aware of the risks inherent in being homeless should initiate appropriate referrals to help patients obtain shelter and thereby reduce their risk of the wide variety of medical problems associated with being homeless, including the risk of trauma. Thus, health workers should play a role in the prevention as well as the treatment of trauma among the homeless.

REFERENCES

1. Alstrom CH, Lindelius R, Salum I. Mortality among homeless men. Brit J Addiction. 1975; 70:245–52.
2. Olin JS. 'Skid row' syndrome: a medical profile of the chronic drunkenness offender. Canad Med Assoc J. 1966; 95:204–14.
3. Buff DD, Kenny JF, Light D. Health problems of residents of single-room-occupancy hotels. NYS J Med. 1980; 80:2000–05.

4. Brickner PW, Greenbaum D, Kaufman, A, et al. A clinic for male derelicts: a welfare hotel project. Ann Int Med. 1972; 77:565–69.
5. Committee on Trauma, American College of Surgeons. Early care of the injured patient. Philadelphia: W. B. Saunders Co., 1982.
6. Greenfield LJ, ed. Complications in surgery and trauma. Philadelphia: J. B. Lippincott Co., 1984.
7. Shires GT. Care of the trauma patient. 2nd edition. New York: McGraw-Hill, 1979.
8. Baxter E, Hopper K. Private lives/public spaces: homeless adults on the streets of New York City. New York: Community Service Society, February 1981.
9. Arce AA, Tadlock M, Vergare MJ, Shapiro SH. A psychiatric profile of street people admitted to an emergency shelter. Hosp and Comm Psychiatry. 1983; 34:812–17.
10. Ropers R, Robertson M. The inner-city homeless: an empirical assessment. Los Angeles: Psychiatric Epidemiology Program, School of Public Health, UCLA, January 1984.
11. Baxter E, Hopper K. The new mendicancy: homeless in New York City. Am J Orthopsychiatry. 1982; 52:393–408.
12. Hopper K, Baxter E, Cox S, Klein L. One year later: the homeless poor in New York City, 1982. New York: Community Service Society, June 1982.
13. Lipton FR, Sabatini A, Katz SE. Down and out in the city: the homeless mentally ill. Hosp and Comm Psych. 1983; 34:817–21.
14. Priest RG. A USA-UK comparison. Proc Roy Soc Med. 1970; 63:441–45.
15. Tenderloin Ethnographic Research Project. Final report. San Francisco: Central City Hospitality House, September 1978.

6

The Problem of Infections: The Experience of the City of Boston's Shelter for the Homeless

John Noble, Thomas Scott,
Laura Cavicci, and Paul E. Robinson

On January 19, 1983, an emergency overnight shelter was established at the Boston City Hospital by ordinance of the Boston City Council. Three months later, the shelter was moved to a dormitory facility at the Long Island Hospital. In its first nine months, the shelter provided overnight lodging to 1150 different people for a total of 23,127 bed-nights, with an average census of 97 people per night.

Medical problems of the shelter's guests have been identified through two surveys: the first conducted on one night during the first week of operation to determine who the guests were; the second based on an analysis of the nursing notes since February 3, 1983. Those who had medical or psychiatric problems and those who required special medications were described in a log book by the nurses on duty. The nursing notes were reviewed for four of the nine months of operation (February, March, August, September) for information on the medical problems encountered among the guests.

INTAKE PROCEDURES

Guests are screened by nurses at Boston City Hospital beginning at 3:00 P.M. each day. Critically ill patients are referred to the emergency room. Each person is searched for weapons, alcohol, and drugs. These individuals then board shuttle buses at 3:45 P.M. and are taken to Long Island Hospital. The guests arrive at 4:00 P.M., and the nurse on duty examines them with the assistance of nurses' aides. Blood pressures are taken, current wounds examined, and medical information and current medications recorded. Medical follow-up care is arranged for as needed. Guests are checked for tuberculosis if there is any indication of its presence, and are then provided with a hot meal and a bed for the night. All guests are required to take a shower, and their clothing is washed. Any guests who may have infestations are treated medically, and all patients are given any medication they may have under nursing supervision.

DEMOGRAPHIC INFORMATION

The average age of the guests at the City of Boston's Shelter for the Homeless is surprisingly young. (See Table 6.1.) Thirty-seven percent are less than thirty years of age; sixty-five percent are forty years of age or younger. Women comprise seventeen percent of the guests, and there were twenty families treated during the first ten months of operation. (See Table 6.2.) A total of 110 children were admitted to the unit during 1983, with ages that ranged from three weeks to nineteen years. At one time, when there were close to 200 patients in the residence, 8 children below the age of five were present.

On the basis of the one-night survey, seventy-three guests gave a recent address in Boston, nine came from other communities in Massa-

Table 6.1. Age Distribution of Guests: City of Boston's Shelter for the Homeless

Age	Percentage
Less than 30 years	37
31–40 years	28
41 and older	35
Total	100

Table 6.2. Guests at the City of Boston's Shelter for the Homeless

Total guests = 1,150
Total bednights = 23,127
Women = 17%
Men = 83%
Families = 20%
Total children (ages 3 weeks to 19 years) = 110
Average census per night = 97 guests

chusetts, and one came from a neighboring New England state. (See Table 6.3.) The birthplaces of the guests reveal more diversity. Twenty-seven were born in Boston, twenty elsewhere in Massachusetts, eight in New England, twenty-four elsewhere in the United States, three outside of the United States, and one who did not know. The educational levels of the guests ranged from eight with elementary school educations, fifty-seven with high school educations, seventeen with college educations, and one guest with a postgraduate degree. (See Table 6.4.) Sixty had been unemployed between one and four years, ten had been unemployed for five to ten years. Thirty-eight stated they could perform skilled work, forty-two unskilled work, and three residents had never been employed. (See Table 6.5.)

MEDICAL EMERGENCIES

In the first nine months, seventy-five medical emergencies were recorded in the shelter, including psychotic episodes, seizures, diabetic reactions, and pregnancy complications. Two patients died of cardiac arrest.

Table 6.3. Residences of Guests: City of Boston's Shelter for the Homeless (one-night survey)

Recent		*Birthplace*	
Boston	73	Boston	27
Massachusetts	9	Massachusetts	20
New England	1	New England	8
Elsewhere in US	0	Elsewhere in US	24
Other	0	Other	3
		Don't Know	1

Table 6.4. Education of Guests (one-night survey)

Elementary	8
High School	57
College	17
Postgraduate	1

A total of twelve seizures occurred in the shelter, and twelve patients required supervised administration of insulin for diabetes mellitus. Three patients awaiting surgery were admitted to the shelter, and one was given lodging while undergoing radiation therapy for carcinoma of the larynx. A total of ten patients were discharged directly from area hospitals to the shelter, and five patients who signed out against medical advice from either hospitals or nursing homes ended up at the shelter. There were eight cases of frostbite and fourteen patients who had to be treated for lice or scabies.

INFECTIONS AMONG THE HOMELESS

Infections common to any group of people gathered close together—such as colds, viral syndromes, and bronchitis—were described by the nurses among the guests at the shelter.

There were two episodes of what appeared to be diarrheal illness. These lasted for only one evening, and food may have been the source. Careful efforts were made to minimize parasitic infestation among the guests. Each guest was carefully examined at intake, and clothes were washed regularly. Whenever a question of lice or scabies arose, patients were immediately given appropriate treatment.

The infections suffered by individual guests fall into four groups: respiratory, gastrointestinal, cutaneous, and musculoskeletal.

Table 6.5. Work History (one-night survey)

Type of Job		Duration of Unemployment	
Skilled	38	1–4 years	60
Unskilled	42	5–10 years	10
Never Employed	3		

Respiratory Illness

Viral illnesses were common. The common cold and sore throat, bronchitis, and viral flu syndromes accounted for 77 percent of all respiratory complaints. (See Table 6.6.) Only three patients were noted to present with what was considered to be a pneumonia. Likewise, there were only three patients who were suspected of having tuberculosis.

Gastrointestinal Illness

Gastrointestinal infections or complaints that might suggest infection are summarized in Table 6.7. Toothache appeared in fifteen guests, stomachache in twelve, gastroenteritis or diarrheal illness in eleven. These patients had significant gastroenteritis as described by the nurse on duty. There were occasionally other patients who complained about diarrhea but were not included in this figure because there were no additional clinical data. Six patients complained of abdominal pain, and most of these required medical referral. One patient stated that he had pancreatitis.

Cutaneous Infections

Cutaneous infections were prevalent among the guests. (See Table 6.8.) Twenty patients had cellulitis, located mostly on the lower extremities. Infected wounds were also a continuing problem at the shelter. Individuals would sustain a wound, receive sutures or treatment at a local hospital, and then, because of neglect or poor care, would develop a secondary infection, which was identified during admission at the shelter. Abrasions were described in twelve patients, contusions in eleven, and lacerations in another eleven. Five patients were referred to the hospital for the treatment of abscesses.

Musculoskeletal Infections

Musculoskeletal afflictions and infections among the guests were concentrated in foot problems (Table 6.9), which were noted forty-three times during the fourth-month record review. The foot problems described are listed in Table 6.10. Trauma, infection, frostbite, and poor-

Table 6.6. Respiratory Infections among Guests (4-month period of observation)

Cold/Sore throat	48
Cough/Bronchitis	21
Viral Flu syndromes	14
Asthma	8
Otitis	5
Conjunctivitis	5
Pneumonia	3
Possible tuberculosis	3
Total	107

Table 6.7. Gastrointestinal Infections among Guests (4-month period of observation)

Toothache	15
Stomachache	12
Gastroenteritis	11
Pancreatitis	1
Abdominal pain	6
Total	45

Table 6.8. Cutaneous Infections among Guests (4-month period of observation)

Cellulitis	20
Infected wounds	12
Abrasions	12
Contusions	11
Lacerations	11
Abscesses	5
Total	71

Table 6.9. Musculoskeletal Infections among Guests (4-month period of observation)

Foot problems	43
Arthritis	24
Leg ulcers	9
Hand problems	5
Total	81

ly fitting shoes produced serious morbidity. Arthritis was present in twenty-four patients, leg ulcers in nine, and problems with the hands in five.

NOSOCOMIAL INFECTIONS

In some instances, infections the guests brought to the shelter were nosocomial in nature. Three preoperative and ten postoperative patients were admitted directly to the shelter following discharge from the hospital. Five of these patients had recently undergone surgical procedures and arrived with dressings and sutures in place. Other patients had infected wounds, which also raised the possibility of nosocomial, as opposed to community-acquired, infections. Poor hygiene and the wide range of ages among the shelter residents increased the possibility of spread of infections.

Guests at the Long Island shelter came from all over Boston. They regularly stayed at other shelters as well and were treated at a wide range of hospitals, described in Figure 6.1. Once at the Long Island shelter, they usually obtained their acute medical care at the Boston City Hospital. This shelter and Boston City Hospital actively related to more than a dozen other health care facilities in eastern Massachusetts. Although there was no evidence for it, nosocomial infections would be easily disseminated as a result of the movement of these individuals throughout the network.

DISCUSSION

This brief review reveals a wide range of infectious problems encountered among guests at the City of Boston's Shelter for the Homeless. Isolated cases and similar problems have been encountered and reported in the epidemiological literature in past years.[1,2] Because of the need to group the guests together in a dormitory-style residence during the cold winter and hot summer months, there was a potential for outbreaks of infectious diseases. Careful bathing and clothes washing procedures appear to have limited the spread of bacterial infections and infestations, although there may have been a spread of upper respiratory viral infections among the guests. The diverse processes by which guests came to the shelter, however, may have lessened the likelihood of identifying epidemics. Each day, almost all of the guests returned to the streets. They then chose whether to return to the Long Island shelter or to spend the following night at another shelter. Among the

Table 6.10. Range of Foot Problems among the Guests

Problems—N = 43 in 4 months
Swelling and/or pain
Rashes
Blisters
Toe ulcers
Tendonitis
Fungal infections
Gunshot wounds
Shoe problems
Frostbite

regular guests, however, there was no evidence of epidemic spread, other than colds and minor upper respiratory illness.

The guests brought with them a wide range of infectious problems, including respiratory, gastrointestinal, cutaneous, and musculoskeletal infections. These infections were noted in 305 residents. If each infection occurred in a different resident, then 26 percent of the residents were affected. We tried to register each resident's problems only once, while surveying the nurses' notes.

The most common infections were relatively minor. They reflected the morbidity profile of illness in a community more than the morbidity profile of an office practice or that of hospitalized populations. The triage system established to check these individuals when they boarded the bus and when they presented themselves at the shelter resulted in the referral of the more seriously ill patients directly to the emergency room at Boston City Hospital.

From these surveys, there appear to have been three types of patients attending the Shelter for the Homeless. A small proportion of patients came with multiple medical problems, including diabetes mellitus, asthma, and frostbite. They were maintained at the shelter for months and required a great deal of nursing care.

The second group of patients were psychiatric and alcoholic patients. Thirty-four percent of the emergency evacuations by ambulance during a three-month period of time were for patients who were acutely psychotic. It has been estimated in another survey of guests at the shelter that 40 percent of the male residents were actively psychotic, and that 80 percent of the female residents were psychotic. The nightly logs record endless conversations with patients who were at best severely disturbed.

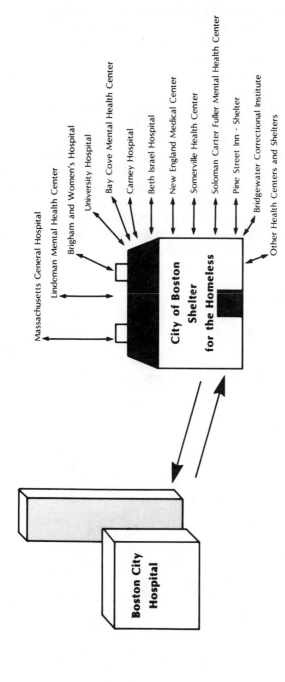

Figure 6.1. Referral Sources of Guests at the City of Boston's Shelter for the Homeless

The final group of residents were those who had planned poorly, had bad luck, or were "down and out": sixteen- and seventeen-year-olds recently evicted from home by their parents, families evicted by landlords, or individuals who came to Boston hoping to find a job before exhausting their money. This group constituted approximately one-third of the residents.

Experience managing infections at the City of Boston's Shelter for the Homeless during nine months in 1983 suggests that consideration should be given to the prevention of outbreaks of infectious disease, the identification of common infectious problems among the guests, and a continuing awareness for the presence of drug-resistant organisms resulting from nosocomial infections. As many as 27 percent of the guests experienced some type of infectious problem while residing at the shelter. While this is a crude estimate, it reflects the prevalence of infectious disease and the importance of this aspect of medical management in shelters for the homeless.

REFERENCES

1. Sherman MN, Brickner PW, Schwartz M, et al. Tuberculosis in single room-occupancy hotel residents: a persisting form of disease. NY Med Quart. 1980; 2:39–41.
2. Rouche B. Eleven blue men. New York: Berkeley Publishing Corp. COP, 1965.

7

Nutritional and Vitamin Deficiency States

Myron Winick

Malnutrition, strictly speaking, is any deviation in the eating pattern of an individual that leads to an abnormal nutritional status. If calorie and protein intake is insufficient, the result is often referred to as protein-calorie malnutrition. This type of malnutrition will cause a series of changes within the body that, if not corrected, can lead to progressive deterioration and death. Fat tissue is completely consumed, muscle mass is markedly reduced, water is lost from the cells and accumulates between them and sometimes within the body's cavities, heart rate slows, blood pressure drops, temperature is subnormal, and the patient responds by doing whatever is necessary to conserve the body's energy. A person suffering from protein-calorie malnutrition shows apathy, slower movements, and decreased activity.

As one of its earliest manifestations, protein-calorie malnutrition will increase an individual's susceptibility to infection by reducing the competence of the immune system. Thus infection, which is very common in the homeless population, could be a complication of, or at least aggravated by, the individual's nutritional status. One important reason to keep the homeless individual's calorie intake as high as possible is to ward off certain kinds of infections rampant in that population.[1]

THE HOMELESS ON THEIR OWN:
VITAMIN DEFICIENCIES

Perhaps much more important than low calorie intake in the homeless in this country is the problem of imbalances: the kinds of foods they eat and the nutrient content of those foods. Insufficient intake of certain vitamins and minerals may lead to specific deficiencies and symptoms caused by those deficiencies. B-vitamin deficiencies can affect the central nervous system; vitamin C deficiency can result in poor wound healing; folic acid, vitamin B_{12}, and iron deficiency can result in anemia; zinc deficiency may cause abnormalities in taste, which in turn may further compromise nutritional status; and calcium deficiency will accelerate the process of osteoporosis, the formation of brittle bones. Many of these deficiencies can be induced by alcoholism.

Most important in the alcoholic are deficiencies of the water soluble vitamins and of certain minerals. We are most concerned about thiamine, vitamin B_6, and folic acid because alcohol interferes with the absorption of all three of these vitamins.[2]

Thiamine deficiency, or beri-beri, is, in the United States, extremely rare in the general population, but it is not uncommon in an indigent alcoholic population. Beri-beri can take two forms. One affects the cardiovascular system and culminates in heart failure. Every resident working in an emergency room must be aware that one cause of high output heart failure in an alcoholic patient is thiamine deficiency. One can cure what we call high output beri-beri by simply giving a shot of thiamine. A second form of beri-beri affects the nervous system: the muscles to the hands and feet weaken and the classical picture of wrist and foot drop results. The homeless, who may have poor nutrition and a high incidence of alcoholism to begin with, are also at risk of thiamine deficiency and the heart failure and neurologic disease that accompany it.

Symptoms of vitamin B_6 deficiency are more insidious and difficult to diagnose. Major deficiencies in vitamin B_6 lead to depression, which is quite common in the homeless populations. The extent to which this depression may be aggravated or induced by a vitamin B_6 deficiency is unknown at the present time.

Folic acid deficiency is the most common vitamin deficiency in the United States. Anybody may be initially presumed as deficient in folic acid. Alcoholics are known to have severe problems with folic acid absorption. Therefore, one would generally predict folic acid deficiency in the homeless.

Folic acid is essential for all cellular division. Thus a deficiency of this vitamin will lead to a slower rate of cell division in those organs where cells are rapidly dividing. The bone marrow, where new blood cells are rapidly being made, is most vulnerable to folic acid deficiency, which leads mainly to a macrocytic type of anemia. It is possible that much of the anemia found in this country's poor is more often due to folic acid deficiency than we tend to believe.

The mineral that we are most concerned about in the poor is zinc, which is also essential for cell division and, therefore, to pregnant women and to children through adolescence. Zinc deficiency can have devastating consequences, including birth defects and poor growth and sexual development. While zinc deficiency in adults is difficult to pinpoint, it leads to two manifestations, each of which could have serious practical considerations. The first are skin rashes, which are common in the homeless person. Second, zinc deficiency leads to abnormalities in taste. Taste is blunted in patients with low levels of zinc in their bodies, and that, too, is a potential problem in the homeless.

Another problem with the homeless is that they are often on drugs (either psychotropic drugs, street drugs, or medications for particular illness), which interact with the diet and can cause certain specific deficiencies. Diuretic drugs may deplete the body's potassium reserves; antiacids may cause an imbalance in the amount of aluminum or magnesium absorbed; aspirin may result in microscopic gastrointestinal bleeding and hence anemia; and many of the so-called tranquilizer drugs can affect appetite.

The classic example is the use of isoniazide for the treatment of tuberculosis. Isoniazide specifically interferes with the metabolism of vitamin B_6, and all patients who are being treated with that drug must be given supplements of vitamin B_6. Dilantin is used in the treatment of epilepsy, yet dilantin interferes with the metabolism of folic acid. Any patient who is being treated with dilantin should be on folic acid supplements. So we see the problems compounded: the same nutrients affected by alcoholism are also affected by certain drugs.[3]

THE HOMELESS UNDER CARE: DIETARY PROBLEMS

Far more important than nutrient deficiencies are the relationships between chronic disease and the kinds of diets these individuals consume. The incidence of hypertension and coronary artery disease is significant among the homeless. And yet if we examine not only what they eat when they are on their own, but what they eat when they are under so-called care, we see that numerous dietary problems persist. These diets are made up from a standard formula prepared by dietitians for institutional patients. Such diets ensure that each of the three meals contains at least one-third of the recommended daily allowance (RDA) for each of the nutrients. The problem is that there are no curbs on the excess of certain nutrients. Because of the epidemic nature of cardiovascular and certain other diseases in this country, Americans should reduce the amount of saturated fat and cholesterol and increase the amount of complex carbohydrate in their diet. In addition, they should reduce the amount of salt or sodium in their diet.[4]

Let us examine a monthly menu schedule. The menu used by the City of New York for its shelter programs provides at least one-third of the daily requirements for all of the known nutrients. However, the menu plan calls for eggs to be served four times a week. Eggs are a very good source of necessary vitamins and minerals, but they are also very high in cholesterol and saturated fat. Cheeses, a commodity that our benevolent government has been giving away, are frequently used. Cheese in general, and particularly hard cheese, is very high in salt (sodium). Lunch or luncheon-type meats such as bologna and hot dogs, which are used frequently, are very high in sodium. Pickled beets, sauerkraut, and sour pickles—again, items served frequently—are also high in sodium.

Not only could such a diet cause problems in people already suffering from hypertension; it could induce hypertension in a population already at high risk. Clearly, we should try to limit the amount of salt and fat in the diet of the homeless population, but there are few attempts to do so. I must commend the imagination of the people in charge of the shelter I visited: much of the snack food they serve comes from AMTRAK, which donates snack food that has not been sold on trains at the end of each day. But while this is an imaginative way of getting food, I wonder how many salty potato chips come from this source.

Another problem, at least in the shelter I visited, was pregnancy. A number of young women were pregnant and homeless. Such a situation imposes major nutritional demands. Weight gain during pregnancy has to be carefully monitored. A pregnant woman, particularly one who comes from a homeless background, should be given supplements or multivitamin and multimineral preparations. She should also be eating foods rich in calcium and iron. This is very difficult, since they are among the most expensive foods on the market. Any woman who is pregnant and homeless is at high risk and probably ought to be hospitalized for a major part of her pregnancy.

The last group at high risk, particularly if homeless, is the elderly, who have specific nutritional needs and requirements. But again, the diets we are giving these people do not reflect those particular needs. One of the major problems in older individuals is osteoporosis.

Osteoporosis is a serious disease. It is the twelfth leading cause of death in the United States and results most commonly in fractures of the vertebrae or hip. Osteoporosis is ten times as frequent in women as in men and is probably the leading cause of serious debility in older women.

Women are more susceptible because they begin to lose calcium from their bones at a relatively rapid rate around age thirty; men do not do this until about age forty. In addition, women increase their calcium demands during pregnancy and lactation. And, finally, further profound changes occur at menopause that result in a dramatic increase in the rate of calcium loss from bones. Low calcium intake aggravates all of these processes. Although the effects of osteoporosis cannot be reversed with calcium, the progression can be slowed. The major source of calcium in the standard shelter diet is milk. But many people cannot tolerate large amounts of milk, due to an inability to digest lactose, or common milk sugar. Lactose intolerance is particularly prevalent in adult blacks and Orientals, as well as in some Caucasians with a Mediterranean background. These people lose most of the activity of the enzyme lactase, which was present in high amounts in childhood. As a consequence, lactose, a disaccharide (carbohydrate made of two sugar molecules), is not split into its compound parts, glucose and galactose. The undigested lactose passes into the lower portion of the gastrointestinal tract, where it is fermented into acids and gases by bacteria, causing diarrhea and gas pain. These symptoms are controlled by reducing the intake of milk and dairy products, thereby avoiding the consumption of lactose.

Thus milk, the food that is richest in calcium content and goes furthest toward providing one-third of the total daily required nutrients in each meal, cannot be consumed by that segment of the population that may need it the most. Substitute foods that are rich in calcium must be found.

The inevitable conclusion is that this population should be given supplementary vitamins and minerals. One must balance risks against benefits. But in balancing the diet and the potential for vitamin deficiency in the homeless against the risk of taking a vitamin preparation,

I believe that this population should receive supplements. This is not being done. Only certain vitamins are sporadically given, subject to availability. Any multivitamin and mineral preparation that provides the recommended daily allowance for each nutrient (not higher) is appropriate.

Thus the homeless population has specific nutritional problems and therefore specific nutritional needs. These are not being met under present conditions, even in the shelter facilities. Perhaps listing these needs, as I have tried to do, will stimulate some change in the way the homeless are fed.

REFERENCES

1. Winick M. Hunger disease: studies by the Jewish physicians in the Warsaw ghetto. Current concepts in nutrition, Winick M, ed., Vol. 7. New York: John Wiley, 1979.
2. Winick M. Nutrition in health and disease. New York: John Wiley, 1980.
3. Winick M. Nutrition and drugs. Current concepts in nutrition, Winick M, ed., Vol. 12. New York: John Wiley, 1983.
4. Winick M. Nutrition and the killer diseases. Current concepts in nutrition, Winick M, ed., Vol. 10. New York: John Wiley, 1981.
5. Winick M. Nutrition disorders in American women. Current concepts in nutrition, Winick M, ed., Vol. 5. New York: John Wiley, 1977.

8

Hypertension: A Screening and Treatment Program for the Homeless

F. Russell Kellogg, Olga Piantieri,
Barbara Conanan, Patricia Doherty,
William J. Vicic, and Philip W. Brickner

Cardiovascular disease is the nation's leading cause of death;[1] and high blood pressure is a major contributor to cardiovascular disease.[2] The nation's most common chronic ailment, hypertension, afflicts an estimated 60 million individuals.[3] Of this number, approximately 35 million need some form of continuing medical treatment and the remaining 25 million, "borderline hypertensives," require ongoing surveillance. Untreated hypertension is the most potent risk factor for stroke and frequently results in heart disease and kidney failure.[4]

In recent years much attention has focused on high blood pressure. Contributing to this heightened awareness were the landmark Veteran's Administration studies,[5,6] which showed that in moderate and severe hypertension, lowering blood pressure through medical treatment results in a marked reduction in mortality and morbidity. More recent work[7] conclusively demonstrated that control of the more common mild forms of hypertension produces a reduced risk of cardiovascular complications. While a few decades ago the goal of treatment

Acknowledgment: the work reported herein was supported in part by a grant from the New York State Department of Health.

was palliation of symptomatic complicated hypertension, early treatment now aims for prevention of these complications through blood pressure control in asymptomatic hypertensives.

Over the past fifteen years significant strides have been made toward achieving this goal.[8] Sustained efforts of government-sponsored programs and professional associations have greatly increased the knowledge base among health professionals as well as the public.[9] These educational efforts, as well as knowledge gained through research, more effective and convenient treatment regimens, and national dietary changes have all helped. Over the last fifteen years we have witnessed a notable reduction in deaths from stroke (42 percent) and heart attacks (25 percent).[10] This decline in hypertension-related mortality is proportionally greater than that seen for noncardiovascular diseases.[10]

Earlier community surveys highlighted the problem of uncontrolled high blood pressure as an unmet public health challenge. Studies from the 1960s and early 1970s reported that half of all hypertensives were undetected, half of those detected were untreated, and half of treated hypertensives were not under satisfactory blood pressure control.[11] Thus, only an estimated 12 percent to 17 percent of hypertensives were under effective treatment. Recent findings of the Hypertension Detection and Follow-up Program[12] indicate that the situation has improved dramatically, to the point that three-quarters of hypertensives are detected, and three-quarters of detected hypertensives are under adequate blood pressure control. Thus, overall, about 40 percent of hypertensives have screening blood pressures below 95 mm Hg diastolic, a decrease of 50 percent or greater compared to figures in earlier surveys.

However, while the national picture has improved overall, certain segments of the population do not appear to have benefited. It has been estimated[13] that perhaps 20 percent of the population is beyond the reach of health care wherein effective management is possible. These medically unreached individuals may suffer the additional disadvantage of an unusually high risk of hypertension because of their racial and behavioral characteristics. Two such groups are the residents of single-room-occupancy (SRO) hotels and the homeless. However, because of the relative inaccessibility of this population to health care and health surveys, exact data about their health problems in general and hypertension specifically are lacking. The few informal surveys reported[14,15,16] do, however, reveal that hypertension and cardiovascular disease are common in the SRO and homeless populations.

Since 1969, the Department of Community Medicine at St. Vincent's Hospital and Medical Center has been involved in efforts to serve medically unreached individuals who are found in temporary shelters and SRO hotels. In November 1983, we established a hypertension control program to improve high blood pressure care in this population.

OBJECTIVES

The goals of our hypertension control program are to:

1. identify all undiagnosed and inadequately treated hypertensive individuals through screening;
2. assure that all identified hypertensives receive an adequate medical evaluation;
3. create and implement a blood pressure control plan for each hypertensive patient that includes both treatment and education; and, finally,
4. assure the continuation of maintenance care directed toward control of blood pressure.

Concurrent with this screening, referral, and treatment program, we are investigating the relationship between alcohol abuse and hypertension.

METHODS

Shelter and SRO residents are screened and rescreened on-site. Participation is voluntary, and methods of recruitment vary depending upon the site. Interviews and blood pressure screenings are done by nurses, physicians, and medical students, all trained and familiar with our protocol for interview and measurement techniques. The interview consists of a general medical history with specific questions about alcohol use and hypertension.

Following the interview, blood pressures are taken and recorded. All blood pressures are taken using a mercury column sphygmomanometer and an appropriately sized cuff, with the individual seated in a quiet environment. Three measurements are taken over a fifteen-minute period. For purposes of blood pressure evaluation, average systolic and diastolic pressures are determined. When the average reading is greater than either 140 mm Hg systolic or 90 mm Hg diastolic, the patient is scheduled to be rescreened at a later date. If the diastolic blood pressure is greater than 120 mm Hg, however, a referral for immediate treatment is made. Individuals with mild or moderate blood pressure elevations are seen again, within several weeks, for repeat blood pressure determinations. If, as before, the average of three consecutive measurements is greater than 140 mm Hg systolic or 90 mm Hg diastolic, a referral is made for a full medical evaluation, usually to our backup hospital clinic. For purposes of this report, all those who had repeated blood pressure elevations are classified "hypertensive." Within our hospital clinic, evaluations include a full medical history and a complete physical examination, an electrocardiogram, chest x-ray, and laboratory screening, all aimed at detecting target organ damage and other cardiovascular risk factors, as well as excluding secondary forms of hypertension.

The specific medical management plan follows an accepted standard protocol.[17] When medications are indicated, a stepped-care approach is used. All patients are advised of nondrug therapeutic measures that will enhance blood pressure control. Follow-up can occur at the SROs and shelters, with periodic clinic visits as needed. Compliance with treatment is closely monitored in all patients.

RESULTS

Between November 1983, and April 1984, we screened 683 individuals at eight sites. (See Table 8.1.) Of the three shelters included, one provided temporary housing for an exclusively female population, one for an exclusively male population, and one for a mixed population. With the exception of one SRO, the hotel population was predominantly male. A large proportion were black and Hispanic. Although many residents in the SROs were middle-aged, one hotel provided housing for a largely elderly population. The age span of the homeless population was broad and included a substantial minority of young individuals.

Table 8.1 depicts the percentage breakdown of the SRO hotel and shelter populations in our study by age, sex and race.

Table 8.1. Demographic Data*

	Age (Years)			Race			Sex	
	45 or less	46–64	65 plus	B	W	H	M	F
Shelter	56	40	4	55	31	14	71	29
SRO Hotel	20	38	42	26	68	6	68	32

*All figures in percentages.

BLOOD PRESSURE FINDINGS

Using the average of three sitting blood pressures on the initial screen and a criterion of greater than 140 mm Hg systolic and/or a diastolic reading greater than 90 mm Hg, we found that, overall, 36 percent of the population surveyed had suspected hypertension. So far, we have been successful in rescreening 96 percent of those who had initial blood pressure elevations and have confirmed the diagnosis in 86 percent of these cases.

The shelter population had an overall hypertension prevalence rate of 28 percent. The majority of individuals screened here were less than forty-five years of age. The SRO population had a 60 percent prevalence rate. Almost half of this population was over sixty-four years of age.

Of the hypertensives identified through interview and screening, a minority were currently under treatment and controlled, others were under treatment but not controlled, a portion were aware of needed treatment but not under care, and a segment were unaware of their problem. (See Table 8.2.)

Analysis of these data indicate that over one-quarter of the people in both groups were unaware of their condition. It appears, however, that a larger proportion of the SRO hotel hypertensives were under medical treatment. While one in four of the SRO hypertensives had controlled blood pressure, the ratio was only about one in ten in the homeless population with hypertension.

The two hypertensive populations were compared by the degree of high blood pressure found, as determined by the initial averaged blood pressure. The proportion of moderate and severe hypertension in the homeless population was almost twice that in the SRO hotel population. (See Table 8.3.)

When we compared the prevalence rates of suspected hypertension in the male subpopulations of heavy regular alcohol users and light or nondrinkers (see Table 8.4), we found that the rate of hypertension among the alcohol-abusing group was at least twice that of the nonabusing group in both the younger and middle-aged males. The differing prevalence rates reached statistical significance despite the relatively small numbers involved ($p < .05$ by chi square analysis).

Thus, these preliminary data suggest that, while a larger proportion of the SRO hotel population had elevated blood pressures, the hypertensives in the shelters were less likely to be under treatment and had more severe hypertension. While interpretation of these data is premature, we may hypothesize that the variance in overall prevalence rates was largely due to age and racial differences in the two populations. It is well documented that the prevalence of hypertension in-

Table 8.2. Hypertensive Groups

	Shelter	SRO
Aware of diagnosis	72%	74%
Currently on treatment	35%	52%
Controlled BP on treatment	11%	24%

creases with age of the population[18] and that blacks have higher rates of hypertension.[19] Thus, because the average age of the SRO residents surveyed was sixteen years greater than that of the shelter population, and the proportion of blacks in the homeless population was twice that of the SRO population, the differing prevalence rates are not unexpected.

That the hypertensives in the shelters were less likely to be under treatment and more likely to have severe hypertension might be explained by factors such as less familiarity with the health care system, greater obstacles to care, and perhaps worse compliance with medical treatment.

That alcohol abuse and hypertension are associated is well known.[20] There is some evidence that heavy alcohol users may suffer three times the rate of stroke as light or nondrinkers.[21] This same study documented that, in a Yugoslavian population, stroke deaths accounted for approximately one-third of the excess mortality suffered by heavy alcohol users. A history of heavy drinking is especially prevalent in stroke patients younger than fifty years of age.[22] Until recently, the nature of the association between alcohol use and hypertension was unknown. Recent published work done by Potter and his colleagues in Great Britain[23] clearly demonstrates the direct "pressor effect" of alcohol in alcohol-dependent hypertensives. Estimates that from 10 percent to as much as 30 percent of so-called essential hypertension may

Table 8.3. Severity of Blood Pressure Elevations (on initial screening)

	Shelter	Welfare Hotel
Controlled on treatment ($<140/90$)	11%	24%
Mild elevation ($>90 < 105$ mm Hg diastolic)	77%	63%
Moderate elevation ($>$ or $= 105 < 115$ mm Hg diastolic)	17%	11%
Severe elevation ($>$ or $= 115$ mm Hg diastolic)	4%	2%

Table 8.4. Male Hypertension Prevalence: Alcohol Abuse and Age

	Age Range (Years)	
	20–34	*35–50*
Current alcohol abuse	33%	44%
No history of alcohol abuse	14%	21%

be due to excessive alcohol consumption places alcohol abuse a close second to obesity as a preventable cause of this disorder.[24]

It appears that hypertension is unusually common in these populations. The reasons for this are not known, but the prevalence of alcoholism and the environmental and psychosocial stresses to which the population are subjected may play a role.

The fact that in both the SRO and shelter populations the vast majority of hypertensives were aware of their condition is somewhat surprising. In fact, the proportion of previously detected "aware" hypertensives is similar to that of the national population.[12]

One might infer that both the SRO and the homeless groups have had significant exposure to the health care system. Indeed, it is our experience that both groups require a great deal of crisis care due to their high incidence of trauma, as well as psychiatric, drug, and alcohol related emergencies. It is common for homeless people to use emergency rooms as their main source of health care.

Despite the fact that the majority of the hypertensives in our survey had been previously detected, only a minority of those identified in the shelter population were currently under treatment at the initial screen. For that population, the proportion under treatment was significantly lower than that found in a recent nationwide survey (35 percent vs. 54 percent).[12] The fraction of SRO residents under treatment was similar to nationwide figures. However, for both populations, the proportion of hypertensives under good blood pressure control was considerably less than that found nationwide (11 percent of shelter hypertensives and 24 percent of SRO hotel residents compared to 38 percent of a nationwide survey).[12] While conclusive interpretation of these figures is hampered by possible selection bias, differing criteria for controlled hypertension, and the demographic mix of our population, it is obvious that the vast majority of hypertensives in both populations were not receiving adequate care.

TREATING THE HOMELESS:
PROBLEMS AND RECOMMENDATIONS

It is highly likely that certain psychological, behavioral, and environmental factors interfere with effective health care for this population. Treatment of hypertension requires ongoing participation by patients in an appropriate setting. It has been documented that episodic emergency room care does not foster good blood pressure control.[25] Certain factors are obstacles to adequate care:

—Intrapsychic factors: Approximately 50 percent of these people have histories of major psychopathology. Many mistrust and fear the health care system.

—Behavioral factors: A substantial minority of these people (about 30 percent) are active alcoholics or drug abusers. Many others pursue very irregular lifestyles, some living day-to-day in a "survival mode." Their disorganized lifestyles impair their ability to make and keep appointments and comply with treatment plans.

—Environmental and social factors: Most lack the social supports that foster good health care. Some health care institutions neglect these people.

—Economic factors: Virtually all of these people are poor. A rising number are becoming homeless because of economic hardship. Our experience indicates that the majority of the homeless population does not have medical insurance coverage. Invariably their choice of foods is based largely upon convenience, cost, or what is available in shelters. Therefore nutritional approaches to treatment are limited.

Any high blood pressure program devised for this population must be prepared to assist the hypertensive patient in overcoming these obstacles. Such a program should:

1. Provide health care professionals who are trained in, and comfortable with, caring for the emotionally disturbed. Also needed are formal psychiatric backup services.

2. Familiarize this team with the management of alcoholism, drug abuse, and the availability of treatment programs for these problems.

3. Provide a substantial proportion of detection, treatment and follow-up services *on-site* at the shelters and SROs where the patients reside.

4. Provide both social support and professional advocacy for those who are sometimes less than welcome at health care institutions.

5. Provide health consultants to the managers of SRO hotels and shelters to make the environments safer.

6. Provide diagnostic services, professional treatment, and medications at no cost to the patient.

7. Maintain ongoing vigilance in follow-up efforts to foster compliance with care.

Our program, using a health team approach with appropriately motivated and experienced professionals, working largely on-site at the shelters and in the SRO hotels and with the full support of our hospital, has met with some initial success. Individuals with confirmed hypertension are referred for medical management and subsequently followed closely by the program team. Of those referred so far, 70 percent have kept their appointments. Of those who are now under treatment, 55 percent have controlled hypertension. While we are enthusiastic about our initial results, we are sobered by the common experience of a high dropout rate among hypertensives in the months following initiation of treatment.[26] Clearly, screening and identifying hypertension is not enough, especially in these populations. Identified hypertensives require appropriate treatment and must be kept under long-term observation.

Is it worth the effort? The magnitude of the problem is clearly significant. In New York City alone, an estimated 36,000 individuals are homeless.[27] If our sample is representative, then approximately 9000 have hypertension and, of these, over 1700 have moderate or severe uncontrolled disease. Without intervention we can predict that many will die or become permanently disabled as a result of cardiovascular complications. We believe that the effort is worthwhile and that useful results can be achieved.

REFERENCES

1. National Center for Health Statistics. Advance report of final mortality statistics, 1981. Monthly Vital Statistics Report, DHHS Pub No (PHS) 84-1120. Pub Health Service, 1984.
2. Kannel WB. Some lessons in cardiovascular epidemiology from Framingham. Am J Cardio. 1976; 37:269.
3. The Joint National Committee on Detection, Evaluation and Treatment of High Blood Pressure. The 1984 report of the joint national committee. Arch Intern Med. 1984; 144:1045.
4. Dawber TR: The Framingham study. Cambridge, Mass.: Harvard University Press, 1980.
5. Veteran's Administration Cooperative Study Group on Antihypertensive

Agents. Effects of treatment on morbidity in hypertension. I. Results in patients with diastolic pressures averaging 115–129 mm Hg. JAMA. 1967; 202:116–22.

6. Veteran's Administration Cooperative Study Group on Antihypertensive Agents. Effects of treatment on morbidity in hypertension. II. Results in patients with diastolic pressures averaging 90–114 mm Hg. JAMA. 1970; 213:1143–52.

7. Hypertension Detection and Follow-up Program Cooperative Group. Five year findings of hypertension detection and follow-up program. I. Reduction in mortality in persons with high blood pressure, including mild hypertension. JAMA. 1979; 242:2562.

8. Moser M. A decade of progress in the management of hypertension. Hypertension. 1983; 5:808.

9. Byington R, Dyer AR, Garside D, et al. Proceedings of the conference on the decline in coronary heart disease mortality. NIH Pub No 79-1610:340. Washington, DC: US Govt Printing Office, 1979.

10. Cooper R, Stamler J, Dyer A, et al. The decline in mortality from coronary heart disease, U.S.A., 1968–1975. J Chuon Dis. 1978; 31:709.

11. Schoenberger JA, Stamler J, Shekelle RB, et al. Current status of hypertension control in an industrial population. JAMA. 1972; 22:559.

12. Wassertheil-Smoller S, Apostolides A, Miller M, et al. Recent status of detection, treatment, and control of hypertension in the community. J Community Health. 1979; 5:82.

13. Kaplan NM. Clinical hypertension. 3rd edition. Baltimore: Williams and Wilkins, 1982:10.

14. Brickner PW, Kaufman A. Case finding of heart disease in homeless men. Bull NY Acad Med. 1973; 49:475.

15. Blumberg L. Skid row and its alternatives. Philadelphia: Temple University Press, 1973.

16. Buff DD, Kenny JF, Light D. Health problems of residents in single room occupancy hotels. NY State J Med. 1980; 80:2000.

17. The 1980 report of the Joint National Committee on detection, education, and treatment of high blood pressure. Arch Intern Med. 1980; 140:1280.

18. Roberts J, Maurer K. Blood pressure levels of persons 6–74 years, United States, 1971–74. Vital Health Stat (11) Series 11. 1977; 203:i–v.

19. U.S. Department of Health, Education, and Welfare, Health Services and Mental Health Administration: Health and nutrition survey 1971–74: advance data: vital and health statistics of the National Center for Health Statistics, no 1. Washington DC: US Govt Printing Office, 1976.

20. Celentano DD, Martinez RM, McQueen DV. The association of alcohol consumption and hypertension. Prevent Med. 1981; 10:590.

21. Kozararevic D, Vojvodic N, Dawber T, et al. Frequency of alcohol consumption and morbidity and mortality. Lancet, 1980; 1:613.

22. Taylor JR. Alcohol and strokes. N Engl J Med. 1982; 306:1111.

23. Potter JF, Beevers DG. Pressure effect of alcohol in hypertension. Lancet. 1984; 1:119.

24. Larbi EB, Cooper RS, Stamler J. Alcohol and hypertension. Arch Int Med. 1983; 143:28.
25. Glass RIM, Mirel R, Hollander C, et al. Screening for hypertension in the emergency department. JAMA. 1978; 240:1973.
26. Wilber JA, Barrow JG. Hypertension, a community problem. Am J Med. 1972; 52:653.
27. Hopper K, Baxter E. Testimony before house committee on banking, finance and urban affairs, subcommittee on housing and community development, December 15, 1982. Washington DC: US Govt Printing Office, 1983:28–39.
28. Manhattan Bowery Corporation. Shopping bag ladies; homeless women. New York, 1979.
29. Baxter E, Hopper K. Private lives/public spaces: homeless adults on the streets of New York City. New York: Community Service Society, 1981.

9

Peripheral Vascular Disease in the Homeless

Kevin McBride and Robert J. Mulcare

Among the diseases afflicting the homeless, leg ulcers, cellulitis, and venous insufficiency have been cited repeatedly. Patch,[1] studying homeless Londoners, estimated 8 percent to be suffering from loco-motor disability. The Manhattan Bowery Project evaluated 200 patients[2] and found that 22 percent of the men were afflicted with dermatological diseases, among which skin ulcers, lacerations, and contusions predominated. A 1973 study[3] reported 41 out of 434 patients, or 10 percent of the study population, to have leg ulcers or cellulitis. In *Mortality Among Homeless Men*, Alstrom[4] found that circulatory problems accounted for four times the number of deaths among that group in Sweden than in the country's general population. At the St. Luke's–Roosevelt Hospital Center of New York City, patients with chronic venous insufficiency and leg ulcers account for about 25 percent of the ambulatory visits to the vascular clinics.

The absolute number of homeless in New York City afflicted with venous stasis disease is unknown. Estimated figures on the number of homeless in the city range from 20,000 to 25,000 men, and 6000 to 7000 women.[2,5,6] Using a conservative figure of 10 percent, based on the previously mentioned studies, an estimated 2600 to 3200 homeless persons suffer from some degree of venous insufficiency. New York City spent about 27 million dollars for the homeless in 1982, a figure that does not include medical expenses. If all of those afflicted were to seek medical treatment for their venous problems at municipal facilities, the additional costs would be significant. In fact, most of the homeless pass transiently through New York's hospitals, both private and public, in time of need and just as rapidly flee the system when temporarily stabilized. Patient compliance as a whole is poor, follow-up difficult, and the living conditions they return to detrimental to good health.

With this background, the present discussion on venous diseases focuses on the methods for ambulatory treatment of homeless patients. The shelter facilities in New York City today offer approximately 4000 beds per night to the homeless. The personnel at these facilities can significantly help those with venous problems by paying attention to the early signs of venous insufficiency and providing basic instruction in dressing changes and hygiene. The most important result to be achieved in this area is the prevention of the complications of venous disease.

PATHOPHYSIOLOGY OF VENOUS ULCERS

Among the peripheral vascular diseases in the homeless, venous disorders of the lower extremities are common. The most prevalent disease in this group is the chronic stasis ulcer. Although many factors contribute to stasis ulcer formation, venous hypertension and a breakdown of local cellular metabolism are the underlying causes.

The etiology of venous hypertension can be traced to a dramatic clinical event, such as deep venous thrombosis, or it can arise from a more insidious cause, like progressive primary valvular incompetence. In either case, the valves in the communicating or perforating branches that bridge the deep and superficial venous systems are destroyed. The result is an increasing column of pressure transmitted down the leg within the superficial venous system. With normal extremities the hydrostatic pressure in the saphenous or superficial system markedly decreases with exercise. The muscular action within the leg increases the flow of blood through the deep veins and increases the drainage of blood from the saphenous system. In the abnormal leg, exercise results in little or no decrease in pressure, due to the reflux of blood back through the deep system after muscular relaxation and an increased passage of blood through the incompetent perforators with muscular contraction. The result is a persistent column of pressure within the legs and a concomitant persistent volume of blood.

The veins dilate and become thickened, and the increased pressure is transmitted to the capillary bed. This alters the permeability of the small venules and capillaries. As a result, there is an accumulation of interstitial fluid and leakage of red blood cells into the tissue surrounding the bed of the superficial veins. This accounts for the clinical signs of edema and hyperpigmentation of the lower extremity.

The metabolic changes at the tissue level are a cellular response to the altered hemodynamic condition. The veins of the lower extremity are more than just conduits for blood. They are an intimate part of the vascular circuit, which provides oxygen and nutrients to the limb and removes metabolic waste products from the local tissue. As a result of increased venous pressure across the capillary bed, tissue oxygen exchange is reduced. Interstitial edema creates osmotic pressure changes in the tissue, altering further the exchange of ions and nutrients across the capillary bed. As oxygen transport is diminished and nutrient exchange reduced, cellular metabolism is altered, with an increase in lactic acid and the breakdown products of anaerobic metabolism. In this respect, the cellular response to venous hypertension is similar to that of peripheral arterial disease. The circulation to an extremity is an intricately balanced network between arteries, capillaries, and veins. The disruption of this balance can lead to hemodynamic abnormalities that result in injury to the local tissue, cell death, and necrosis. Since the area most affected by venous hypertension is the tissue surrounding the saphenous system, tissue necrosis from venous statis ulcers tends to be superficial, usually external to the fascial level. Necrosis commonly involves the lower medial third of the leg, following the distribution of the saphenous system, and may produce wide and irregular ulcers, which exude significant amounts of interstitial fluid.

Our experience in the outpatient facilities and emergency room at St. Luke's–Roosevelt Hospital in New York includes treatment of large numbers of patients with venous ulcers. From the clinical point of view, several common medical histories are communicated by homeless patients brought to medical attention. One such history is that of the postphlebitic syndrome. Patients describe an occasion in the past when one of their legs became painfully swollen, usually around the calf but sometimes as high as the thigh. They may have been hospitalized at that time, or weathered the acute inflammation in a dorm or shelter until they could walk again. This was the period of deep venous thrombosis. They further explain that, since the original episode, the affected leg seems to be larger than the other and swells each day. By nightfall, when they retire, the ankle and lower leg ache and their shoes no longer fit as they used to. Clearly, during this period venous hypertension is present and edema formation has occurred. Lastly, they will usually recount that more recently the swollen leg has become itchy and the skin seems to flake around areas of the rash. This dermatitis and eczema associated with chronic venous insufficiency is the preterminal phase before frank tissue loss and ulceration.

A similar history, but without an acute event such as deep venous thrombosis, concerns progressive valvular incompetence. These patients usually describe progressive swelling, which is worse when they rise in the morning, of either one or both lower extremities. The history may point to the fact that certain homeless people sleep in a sitting position, semiupright and flexed at the waist, on park benches or in cramped spaces. This position causes plupiologic—that is, gravitational—and mechanical outflow obstruction to the deep venous system and requires higher venous pressures to return the blood to the heart. Over a prolonged period of time, these higher pressures result in progressive valvular destruction as the blood attempts to find alternate paths, such as through the superficial system, to reach the heart. Eventually, the outcome is progressive edema, hyperpigmentation, inflammation, and ulceration.

The development of venous stasis ulcers, although a matter not unique to the homeless, presents particular problems to these people and their lifestyle. Once an ulcer has formed, the barriers to infection are broken down. The loss of skin integrity and the exposure of subcutaneous tissue to the surface allows for contamination of the deep tissue by the bacteria that characteristically inhabit the skin. Organisms such as staphylococcus and streptococcus species, normally found on healthy skin, can invade an ulcer and cause localized cellulitis. The organisms cultured from infected ulcers are not restricted to these gram-positive cocci. *Hemophilus influenzae* and a host of other gram-negative bacilli have been found frequently in chronic stasis ulcers with and without cellulitis. Infected ulcers require prompt medical attention; they pose a significant threat to life or limb. The lifestyle of the homeless increases the likelihood that stasis ulcers will become infected and thus more serious. It is important to these people to identify early signs of venous stasis disease, before frank ulceration occurs. Teaching shelter staff and homeless people who pass through shelters to recognize the hallmarks of venous diseases should certainly help prevent ulcers. Access to facilities where early diagnosis can delay or prevent some of the complications of venous hypertension, and the use of existing techniques to aid that diagnosis, is also important.

NONINVASIVE TESTING

In the vascular laboratory several noninvasive methods have been developed to assess acute and chronic venous disease. The Doppler flowmeter described by Rushmer and his colleagues[7] measures blood flow. A small probe produces ultrasound at a particular frequency that red blood cells moving through reflect back to a transducer in the same probe. The change in frequency is proportionate to the flow. One can listen to the flow rates in both the deep and superficial venous systems. Strandness[8] was among the first to describe the use of ultrasound for the diagnosis of venous disease. Application of various compression cuffs above and below the site where the Doppler probe is held can indicate whether the valves in either system are competent. These sounds are both audible and capable of being recorded on paper. Although this technique is not 100 percent accurate, it is a simple, inexpensive screening device, particularly for recent thrombosis involving the femoral and popliteal veins above the knee.

Plethysmography is another noninvasive technique that has been extensively used for the diagnosis of venous disease.[9-12] In our laboratory, the photoplethysmography technique is employed. A tiny photocell is placed on the skin of the lower leg. The cell emits an infrared signal that reflects off the tissues under the cell. The reflected signal, which is proportional to the flow under the probe, is received in a transducer and recorded. The patient exercises for five seconds with the photocell strapped to the leg, emptying the venous system of a significant portion of its blood volume. The time the blood takes to return to preexercise levels is a determinant of venous insufficiency. Normal individuals will refill the venous system via their arterial inflow, passing from artery to capillary and finally into the veins; this may take perhaps twenty-five to thirty seconds. The patient with incompetent valves may refill the system in three to five seconds due to the reflux effect of venous blood passage across the destroyed valves.

None of these methods for detecting deep vein thrombosis or chronic venous insufficiency are perfect; but they have the advantage of being inexpensive and noninvasive. They can be performed rapidly in an outpatient setting and are suitable as a screening procedure for people suspected of venous disease. Patients such as the homeless, who may suspect problems with their legs or who have been noted by workers in the dorm or shelter to have early signs of venous stasis, could be easily tested in an outpatient medical setting before ulcers and their complications set in.

TREATMENT

The treatment of venous stasis disease is twofold. The first approach should be directed toward relieving the problems of venous hypertension and pooling in persons with chronic venous insufficiency. Methods to reduce ambulatory venous pressure in the lower legs must be utilized daily to achieve effective control. The second area of treatment addresses the problem of care for the existing venous ulcer; simple guidelines need strict observance if healing is to occur.

The most basic aid for patients with chronic venous stasis is recumbency with leg elevation. When the supine leg is raised above the level of the heart, gravity will assist in drawing blood from the legs to the pelvis, and back to the heart. Leg elevation from a horizontal position can diminish ambulatory venous pressure a hundredfold relative to standing and approximately tenfold relative to sitting. Placing one or two pillows or blankets beneath the calves when the patient is supine during the night will serve the purpose. Elevation alone can dramatically decrease swelling (edema) in the feet, ankles, and calves of patients with venous insufficiency. Most individuals can start the day with minimal edema, thus reducing the degree of eczematous change and inflammatory reaction that occurs with persistent swelling.

Once the person is on his or her feet during the day, the edema will recur and the ankles will swell again. Therefore the ambulatory person, homeless or otherwise, needs treatment with external compression devices. The use of elastic stockings as external support for the treatment of venous insufficiency has been well documented.[13-15] External compression stockings have been shown to increase mobilization of blood from dependent parts of the lower extremity, reduce venous reflux in incompetent veins, and increase the period of volume reduction after exercise to values approaching normal controls.[15] These stockings range from simple commercial brands found in shoe and clothing stores, with modest compressive effectiveness, to individually measured and fitted stockings, with proven benefit. The stockings should be worn throughout the course of the day, and removed when the patient retires for the night. Ill-fitted stockings can produce pressure lines or constrictive cuff markings that are potentially detrimental and are to be avoided. External compression stockings bought in standard sizes and distributed through the shelter to homeless individuals with documented venous insufficiency may prove cost-effective by reducing the rate of ulcer formation and its more expensive treatment.

When frank ulceration does occur, a more concentrated treatment plan, requiring a higher compliance by the affected individual, must begin. Daily washing of the ulcer with simple soap and water is a basic necessity to prevent infection. Legs should be kept clean. Use of dry laundered socks can help minimize microtrauma to the affected leg and reduce the spread of further ulcerations.

Most ulcers arise near the ankle, in the area of the medial malleoli.[16] They often develop in areas of induration and dermatitis. When stasis dermatitis is manifested by itching and flaking skin with weeping edematous areas, topical antibiotic therapy has proven efficacious. After cleansing the leg in lukewarm water, topical ointments may be applied, such as polymyxin B-bacitracin (Polysporin®), polymyxin B-bacitracin-neomycin (Neosporin®), erythromycin (Ilotycin®), or gentamicin sulfate (Garamycin®).[17] These antibiotic ointments should be applied daily, then covered with dry dressings and compressive wraps such as Ace bandages.

In many medical centers an alternative approach to daily dressing changes has been employed with good results. Patients with stasis ulcers that are not secondarily infected can benefit from the application of an Unna boot dressing. The Unna boot is a prepackaged bandage roll impregnated with a paste of zinc oxide, calamine, glycerin, and gelatin. It is applied to the foot and lower leg and can remain on the extremity for up to one week. A loosely applied Ace wrap over the dressing can help protect the medicated bandage from external contamination. The directions for applying the Unna boot are well illustrated on the package, and the relative infrequency of changes is a particular benefit to the ambulatory and homeless population. This boot not only provides a practical medicated dressing to the skin, but also gives external support, which reduces the local venous pressure and underlying stasis. The cost-effectiveness of such a treatment plan can only be measured against the background of patient compliance, ease of application, number of dressing changes necessary, and total cost created by this chronic disease and its more serious complications.

When secondary infection has developed from a leg ulcer with cellulitis, lymphangitis, or septicemia, the patient must be referred to a medical facility. Systemic antibiotic therapy, bedrest, elevation, and wound debridement should be instituted promptly. In-hospital treatment must continue until the infection has cleared and the cellulitis has resolved. Patients with chronic ulcers who fail to respond to repeated conservative therapies are advised to seek a surgical referral for skin grafting.

DIABETIC FOOT ULCERS

Several important points should be stressed with regard to patients with diabetes mellitus. First, diabetic patients are much more susceptible to infection than the normal population. Small cuts or trauma to toes or heels can result in rapidly spreading infection with possible life-threatening consequences. Second, many diabetics develop a neuropathy that can manifest itself as a painful foot or one with diminished or absent sensation. Thus ambulatory diabetics with neuropathy may develop pressure sores or trauma to parts of the foot and be unaware of the injury until infection has spread through the extremity and into the circulation. Third, diabetics frequently develop peripheral vascular occlusive disease. Unlike the nondiabetic pattern of atherosclerosis, diabetics suffer more from small artery disease. This usually involves the distal arteries of the leg and foot, where calcification and obstruction can lead to ischemic digits, or skin ulcers of the foot. Any ulcer of the foot, infection, or sore seen in a homeless diabetic patient requires immediate referral to a medical facility. The consequences of delay are far too devastating to risk suboptimal treatment of these patients. This, combined with the lifestyle of a homeless person, could result in loss of life or limb if improperly treated.

REFERENCES

1. Patch ICL. Homeless men in London. Br J Psychiatry. 1971; 118:313–17.
2. Shopping bag ladies; homeless women. New York: Manhattan Bowery Corporation, 1979.
3. Brickner PW, Kaufman A. Case finding of heart disease in homeless men. Bull NY Acad Med. 1973; 49(6):475–84.
4. Alstrom CH. Mortality among homeless men. Br J Addictions. 1975; 70: 245–52.
5. U.S., Congress, House, Committee on Banking, Finance, and Urban Affairs, Subcommittee on Housing and Community Development, testimony of Hopper K and Baxter E. Washington, DC: US Govt Printing Office, 1983:28–39.
6. Baxter E, Hopper K. Private lives/public spaces: homeless adults on the streets of New York City. New York: Community Service Society, 1981.

7. Rushmer RF, Baker DW, Stegall HF. Transcutaneous Doppler flow detection as a non-destructive technique. J Appl Physiol. 1966; 21:554.

8. Strandness DE, Schultz RD, Sumner DS, Rushmer RF. Ultrasonic flow detection: a useful technique in the evaluation of peripheral vascular disease. Am J Surg. 1967; 113:311.

9. Wheeler HB, Mullick SC. Detection of venous obstruction in the leg by measurement of electrical impedance. Ann NY Acad Sci. 1970; 170:804.

10. Johnston KW, Kakkar VV. Plethysmographic diagnosis of deep vein thrombosis. Surg Gyn Obst. 1974; 137:44.

11. Yao ST, Needham TN, Gourmoos C, Irvine WT. Plethysmography and Doppler ultrasound in arterial disease of the lower extremities. Surgery. 1972; 71:4.

12. Darlwig RC, Raines JK, Brenner BJ, Austin WG. Quantitative segmental pulse volume recorder: a clinical tool. Surgery. 1972; 72:873.

13. Sigel B, Edelstein AL, Felix WR, Menhardt CR. Compression of the deep venous system of the lower leg during inactive recumbency. Arch Surg. 1973; 106:38.

14. Somerville JJF, Brow GO, Byrne PJ, et al. The effect of elastic stockings on superficial venous pressures in patients with venous insufficiency. Surgery. 1974; 61:979.

15. Gjores JE, Thulesius O. Compression treatment in venous insufficiency evaluated with foot volumetry. Vasa. 1977; 6:364–68.

16. Schwartz S, ed. Principles of surgery. New York: McGraw-Hill, 1979.

17. Young JR. Thrombophlebitis and chronic venous insufficiency. Geriatrics. 1973; 28:63–69.

10

Alcoholism and the Homeless

Robert Morgan, Edward I. Geffner,
Elizabeth Kiernan, and Stephanie Cowles

Twenty years ago, in the face of differing opinions, the American Medical Association felt compelled to acknowledge alcoholism as a disease.[1] Prior to this time, except by a few committed organizations and individuals, alcoholism was generally regarded as a form of indulgence and alcoholics were seen as moral degenerates rather than sick people in need of treatment.[2] This attitude was manifested and reinforced by laws against public drunkenness and a marked lack of therapeutic resources for chronic alcoholics.[3]

Historically in the United States, public intoxication was managed through the penal system.[3] In New York State, for example, laws concerning public inebriates appeared on the books in the early 1800s and by 1833 public intoxication was outlawed altogether.[4] New York State's use of the criminal justice system to manage public inebriates was typical of the rest of the country.

Just prior to World War II and in the two decades immediately thereafter, alternate views on the nature and treatment of alcoholism developed, culminating in the establishment of the National Institute on Alcohol Abuse and Alcoholism (NIAAA) and the passage of legislation that decisively changed society's treatment of alcoholics and al-

coholism.[2,5-7] A series of federal court decisions that addressed the
question of criminal culpability for public inebriation illustrates that
change. In *Easter* v. *District of Columbia* [316 F. 2d 50 (D.C. Cir., 1966)]
and *Driver* v. *Hinnant* [356 F. 2d 761 (4th Cir., 1966)], two circuit courts
declared that public inebriates were sick people akin to lepers or the
mentally ill. These courts declared that criminal prosecutions of public
drunkenness ran afoul of the Eighth Amendment's prohibition against
cruel and unusual punishment and required proof of intent to commit
a prohibited act for a finding of guilt. These cases were litigated by attorneys on behalf of the American Civil Liberties Union (ACLU) and
the Washington Area Council on Alcoholism. In a similar case, *Powell*
v. *Texas* [392 U.S. 514 (1968)], Leroy Powell, represented by the same
ACLU attorneys who tried the *Easter* and *Driver* cases, went to the
Supreme Court to challenge the constitutionality of jailing chronic
alcoholics, again based on the Eighth Amendment. In a five-to-four decision, the Justices found that chronic alcoholics appeared drunk in
public under a compulsion symptomatic of the disease of alcoholism,
but they nevertheless did not accept the disease as a defense to the
crime of public drunkenness and upheld Powell's conviction. Although
troubled by the issue, Justice Marshall, who wrote the majority opinion,
concluded that it was rational to use the criminal process to cope with
the public aspects of problem drinking. The Court based its decision
on the fact that doctors disagreed about both the concept of alcoholism
as a disease and the nature, degree, and methods of treatment. Further, in light of inadequate treatment facilities, the Court considered
jails useful in removing alcoholics from the streets and providing them
with a place to dry out. Nonetheless, the criticism levied in the Court's
majority and minority opinions against the lack of treatment programs
and the fears and prejudices that infected the public's perception of alcoholics lent a powerful thrust to efforts that eventually resulted in decriminalization of public intoxication in some states and the development of therapeutic alternatives to jail.

The *Powell* case called into question the extent to which the medical
profession accepted the definition of alcoholism as a disease, allowed
by the *Easter* and *Driver* courts. However, this case made clear what
a poor substitute the traditional system of jailing drunks was for humane medical treatment. The system was in jeopardy and new alternatives were urgently needed.

Saint Louis, Missouri, was the first city in the United States to establish a detoxification program.[3] It was housed in a former obstetrical
hospital, and used a medical model. The program offered public inebriates five to seven days of treatment. Librium® was used to sedate

patients during the withdrawal process. After detoxification, patients were referred for further treatments, usually to halfway houses.[3]

Although treatment at the Saint Louis Project was voluntary, the men were under a great deal of pressure to enter and remain in the program. The patients brought in by the police were given the option of going to the detoxification center or to jail. Each patient received a physical exam and was cared for by nurses and physicians, while a social worker planned further treatment. A patient who chose to sign out before the detoxification period was up was issued a summons.[8]

In 1966, after the *Driver* and *Easter* decisions, the City of New York invited the Vera Institute of Justice to develop a medically oriented method for removing destitute alcoholics from the streets. Unlike the Saint Louis Project, Vera decided on a genuinely voluntary program that would not resort to jail in cases where treatment failed.[9,10]

One year later, Vera created the Manhattan Bowery Project (MBP), a free-standing medical detoxification program designed to provide short-term treatment for Bowery alcoholics.[9,10] The Project's rescue team sought out distressed alcoholics and offered them a chance to detoxify in a safe, warm place. The overwhelmingly positive response to voluntary detoxification quickly dispelled the myth that Bowery men preferred drinking to treatment. However, it soon became apparent that medical detoxification alone did not provide a cure for alcoholism and that long-term rehabilitation programs were needed. This awareness caused MBP to devise a more comprehensive spectrum of treatment services that included an outpatient department, two residential treatment programs, a halfway house, and a nonmedical detoxification unit.[10] The Bowery experiment was so successful as an alternative to criminal justice processing that it eventually led to the decriminalization of public intoxication in New York State on January 1, 1976.[10,11]

Federal legislation further stimulated the general shift toward decriminalization of public drunkenness. The award of federal dollars for treatment was tied to the enactment of decriminalization statutes by the states.[12] The fund was administered by the National Institute on Alcohol Abuse and Alcoholism (NIAAA), the new agency established to promote the treatment of alcoholism.[13] These developments brought about a dramatic change in public and professional perspectives on alcoholism. The disease concept is now firmly established, and growing numbers of professionals are involved in treatment services.[14-16] In several states there are reasonably adequate resources to provide care for all alcoholics regardless of income.[17] At this writing, thirty-three states have decriminalized public intoxication.[18]

However, the picture is not perfect. The controversy over whether to jail or treat public inebriates continues. Even in some states that have decriminalized public intoxication, workers in the field disagree about whether compulsion—the use of the police—is necessary to induce skid row alcoholics to accept treatment.[19-22] Moreover, knowledge of the etiology and treatment of alcoholism is in its infancy. An enormous amount of work remains to be done to determine the biochemical and psychological processes that cause alcoholism and to improve the effectiveness of treatment of this disease and its medical complications.[23]

ALCOHOLISM

According to the United States Public Health Service, alcoholism, a chronic, progressive disease, is one of this country's ten major health problems, affecting some ten million people.[24] Alcoholism is defined as the ingestion of more than 80 gm of alcohol daily for more than five years. The daily amount is equivalent to six one-and-one-half-ounce drinks of whiskey, six cans of beer, or six four-ounce glasses of wine.

Often alcoholism is unrecognized or deliberately ignored by patient and doctor because of the stigma it carries. There have been estimates that anywhere from 15 to 40 percent of all hospitalized persons are admitted because of alcohol-related problems. Nevertheless, this diagnosis is often not recorded:[25,26] many medical insurance plans do not cover treatment for this disease.

In addition to the social deterioration that accompanies alcoholism, every system of the body is or can be touched by the disease process.[27] In alcoholism's earlier stages, the diagnosis cannot always be clearly made. In the absence of rapid social deterioration and moderate-to-severe withdrawal symptoms, the fledgling alcoholic is often misdiagnosed. Since denial is a part of the disease process of alcoholism, the patient often thwarts its diagnosis.

Although the etiology of alcoholism is not known, genetics seems to play a role.[25,28] It appears from recent family studies that people have a greater chance of becoming alcoholic if one or both parents has had the disease.[29]

Alcoholism is both progressive and chronic. In its first stage it is characterized by an increase in alcohol tolerance. The individual drinks to relieve tension or anxiety and begins to drink in secret. There is an urgency associated with obtaining the first drink of the day. In the second stage, the alcoholic begins to feel guilty about drinking, but tolerance of and physical dependence on alcohol increases. A person who has advanced to full-blown third-stage alcoholism will find it very difficult to maintain sobriety even for a short time because of the strong physical dependence.[30] The alcoholic when sober experiences a strong craving for a drink and seems unable to feel normal, much less tranquil, without it. After taking a drink or two the alcoholic feels "good" for an hour or two, after which time the alcohol's effect wears off and a slight withdrawal reaction begins. The drinker feels a little worse than before the first drink, with a craving for more and the need to ease the withdrawal. In this way a long-term binge begins.

Withdrawal is characterized by increased heart and pulse rate, tremors, sweating, a general feeling of anxiety and distress, and, in more severe cases, elevated temperature and blood pressure readings. The severity of the reaction will vary with the degree of intoxication and the length of time during which a person has been drinking before stopping. Thus a person who has averaged a few drinks a week will have a very mild, all but unnoticeable, reaction, while a chronic skid row alcoholic may experience violent tremors, seizures, or even full-blown delirium tremens.

THE HOMELESS ALCOHOLIC

Although alcoholism strikes all classes of people, regardless of sex, age, race, or economic status, the most common image of an alcoholic remains the public inebriate or skid row alcoholic.[2] For many years homelessness and chronic alcoholism were virtually synonymous.[31-34]

Estimates in alcoholism literature are consistent in stating that 3 to 5 percent of the ten million alcoholics in the United States are on skid row.[35] In 1982 the Community Service Society drew a statistical profile of the men in New York City's public shelter system, using data from five different studies commissioned by the city's Human Resources Administration (HRA).[36] Although only 14 percent of the men attributed their arrival at or return to emergency shelters to drinking, on clinical examination nearly 25 percent showed evidence of alcohol dependency.[37,38] Today, alcoholics are recognized as a subset of the homeless population, although the exact percentage is not known.[39]

There are several ways to estimate the alcoholic skid row population. The HRA study cites an estimated 5600 to 10,000 homeless alcoholics. The Manhattan Bowery Corporation (MBC) admits some 2000 different individuals to their detoxification programs each year,[10] while other detoxification programs in the city serve an additional 7000 patients annually. These figures would indicate at least 9000 skid row alcoholics in New York City. A third method of estimation assumes that 3 to 5 percent of the alcoholics in New York City are public inebriates. This would mean there are 15,000 to 25,000 such individuals.[40] Thus the range of public inebriates in New York City, derived from all three methods, is anywhere from 5600 to 25,000. The higher numbers are believed to be more accurate, since it is unlikely that all public inebriates receive detoxification program services.

Less clear and more difficult to quantify is the degree of alcoholism and alcohol abuse among the emotionally disturbed homeless, the young runaways, the elderly poor, destitute families, and other victims of poverty. Those who work with these populations guess the percentage of alcoholics and alcohol abusers to be anywhere from 15 to 35 percent.[41,42]

Whatever their number, these people are the most difficult to reach and treat and present a host of problems associated with extreme poverty that do not occur in middle class populations.[25,43] Moreover, public inebriates are often in the late stage of alcoholism and may suffer from a variety of medical problems associated with this advanced condition.

According to sociologist Earl Rubington, who has contributed much to the literature concerning the skid row alcoholic, the recovery rate among this group is a great deal lower than the success rate among alcoholics from the general population being treated in average programs.[44,45] Despite this lower rate of success, the experience of the Manhattan Bowery Corporation and other programs for public inebriates indicates that homeless alcoholics can be treated for their disease and are willing to come for treatment.[10,46]

The skid row alcoholic has settled on drinking to get through the day, a day often filled with tension. Although the alcohol precipitates the disease to the point of homelessness on skid row, life on the street strongly reinforces the urge to drink and often interferes with efforts to stop.

Although many alcoholics have chronic diseases such as epilepsy, diabetes mellitus, or cardiac disability, they will often miss clinic appointments and lose or fail to take medicine because their sole interest is in drinking. Moreover, cerebral atrophy from chronic alcoholism or multiple head injuries over the years may further cloud judgment and capacity to take personal responsibility. Thus, while skid row alcoholics who come to emergency rooms or detox units most often present withdrawal symptoms, they may also be in a deteriorated state from diseases affecting many organs.[47]

MEDICAL COMPLICATIONS
OF ALCOHOLISM

The medical complications of alcoholism are numerous, leaving few parts of the body untouched. Primary complications are those affecting the *nervous system*, the *gastrointestinal system*, the *liver*, the *pancreas*, and the *heart*. And the condition termed "fetal alcohol syndrome" can affect the unborn child of a female alcoholic.

An estimated 50 to 70 percent of sober skid row alcoholics in treatment have central *nervous system* dysfunction.[48] Long-term heavy drinking often results in brain atrophy, accompanied by enlargement of the ventricles and widening of the sulci. Recent investigations using computerized tomography (CAT) brain scans and pneumoencephalograms indicate that brain damage may precede liver injury and be of far greater importance.[49,50] However, contrary to earlier opinion, at least partial recovery of the brain from atrophy has been demonstrated by CAT scans done months after abstinence or diminished drinking.[51]

The Wernicke syndrome, a thiamine deficiency disease caused by alcoholic drinking, is a state of global confusion, ophthalmoplegia, nystagmus, and ataxia. More than 80 percent of skid row alcoholic patients also show peripheral neuritis, while postmortem pathological examination shows altered neural structures in the subcortical areas of the cerebellum and brain stem.[42] Wernicke's syndrome is a medical emergency. If not treated with high doses of thiamine, the disease may end in death.[28,52]

Most of those who recover from Wernicke's syndrome are left with a longstanding Korsakoff's syndrome: amnesia for recent events with confabulation and a passive, indifferent personality. Only 20 percent recover completely. The residual state includes large gaps in memory without confabulation and the inability to sort events in their proper temporal sequence.

The peripheral nervous system, involving motor and sensory nerves to the extremities, suffers axonal degeneration due to nutritional deficiency and the direct toxic effect of alcohol.[53] The consequent numbness, tingling, and unsteady gait often respond well to or are cured completely by good nutrition and abstinence from alcohol.

Dysfunctions of the *gastrointestinal system* are common among alcoholics. Patients with bleeding esophageal varices, mucous membrane tears at the gastroesophageal junction, and hemorrhage from the stomach due to alcohol gastritis are well known to hospital emergency room staff.[54] Although fiberoptic endoscopy can identify the source of the hemorrhage precisely, its use is not associated with improved mortality figures.

Gastritis has been found in 25 percent of alcoholics admitted for detoxification.[55] Ethanol disrupts the gastric mucosal barrier, producing a back diffusion of hydrogen into the cell. This causes swelling and exfoliation and with prolonged alcohol use leads to erosions and hemorrhage.[56,57]

Cirrhosis of the *liver* is the third leading cause of death in urban males in the United States, and the main cause is heavy alcohol abuse.[58] Leevy found a 30 percent incidence of cirrhosis in liver biopsies of 3000 heavy drinkers.[59]

Ninety percent of ingested alcohol is metabolized to acetaldehyde in the liver. Here alcohol dehydrogenase transfers hydrogen from alcohol to nicotinamide adenine dinucleotide (NAD), forming NADH. This hydrogen is then used by the liver mitochondria as a preferential energy source instead of the hydrogen from fat, the usual energy source. Therefore fat accumulates in the liver, augmented by endogenous fat formation and increased fat transport from peripheral adipose tissue throughout the body. The swollen fatty liver cells in some cases become inflamed with polymorphonuclear cells. First necrosis, then cirrhosis, develops, due to increased collagen formation in the liver from fibroblast activity. [60]

The diagnosis of cirrhosis is made by liver biopsy. The tissue shows increased scarring and microtubular regeneration. The disease is well recognized clinically by the complications of ascites, portasystemic encephalopathy, jaundice, bleeding esophageal varices, abnormal blood coagulation, body wasting, and finally death. This disease is entirely preventable by abstinence from alcohol. For those who continue to drink, the five-year survival rate is 40 percent once the diagnosis of cirrhosis is made; but abstinence will increase the five-year survival rate to 63 percent.[61]

The *pancreas*, too, is adversely affected by alcohol. After many years of drinking, especially if it is accompanied by a high-fat or high-protein diet, the protein components of the pancreatic juice combine with calcium to form substances that obstruct the pancreatic ducts. The consequence is acute and chronic abdominal pain, glucose intolerance, pancreatic digestive insufficiency, and possibly pseudocysts of the pancreas. Methods of abating this condition work poorly, especially for the pain syndrome. Apart from analgesia and abstinence from alcohol, there is little that medical management can offer for patients with pain of chronic pancreatitis.

Fetal alcohol syndrome occurs in about one-third of the infants born to women who drink five ounces or more of alcohol per day during pregnancy.[12] It is characterized by small head circumference, mental retardation, and cardiac and joint abnormalities. The precise mechanism by which this disorder develops is unknown.

Finally, alcoholism is associated with *heart* problems. Heavy drinkers may have arrythmias or depressed myocardial function. The term "holiday heart" has been applied to intermittent arrythmias associated with weekend drinking.[63] Alcoholic cardiomyopathy may be due to thiamine deficiency or to direct toxic effects of alcohol on the heart. Hypertension is not affected by moderate use of alcohol, but for users of two and one-half ounces or more of pure alcohol per day, its prevalence is double that for the population at large.[64]

TREATMENT AND PROGRAM GOALS

The homeless alcoholic presents a number of concrete clinical problems to treatment personnel. These are due in part to poverty and in part to the advanced state of the patient's alcoholism, characterized by lengthy periods of intoxication that end only when the alcoholic is too ill to continue drinking and by feelings of hopelessness regarding the ability to live without alcohol.[65]

Entering Treatment

The public inebriate's first contact with alcoholism treatment is often admission to a detoxification unit, where withdrawal from alcohol occurs under observation. The withdrawal process causes tremors, insomnia, hyperarousal, and anxiety. And contrary to popular belief, it is more dangerous than withdrawal from heroin. In severe cases the patient will have convulsions, seizures, alcoholic hallucinosis, and full-blown delirium tremens. The motivation to detox is the physical inability to continue the drinking episode, whether because of the severity of gastritis, lack of money to buy alcohol, or other reasons.

There are two appropriate detoxification methods for the homeless alcoholic: inpatient medical detoxification, in which the staff administers medication that alleviates withdrawal symptoms; and nonmedical detoxification, which relies on environmental manipulation rather than medication to lessen the physical effects of alcohol withdrawal.[66-68] Ambulatory detoxification, in which a physician prescribes withdrawal medication for a detoxification regimen to an outpatient, is not suitable, since it requires a stable and supportive home environment for success.[69]

Medical Detoxification

A medical detoxification unit uses minor tranquilizers or sedative hypnotics to control withdrawal symptoms.[25] On admission to a medical unit, the alcoholic is seen by a nurse and a physician, who take a medical history, conduct a physical examination, and order laboratory tests and, if indicated, x-rays. The withdrawal regimen for the alcoholic usually involves sedatives, anticonvulsant medications, vitamins, minerals, and antacids. If indicated by the intake screening, the physician will also order treatment for other illnesses. Alcoholism counselors meet with the client on several occasions to discuss the disease and offer referral to either an inpatient or outpatient alcoholism treatment program. The counseling staff also addresses any social, medical, and work-related needs the patient may have and conducts therapy groups and alcoholism education seminars.[70]

Nonmedical Detoxification

Nonmedical detoxification relies on a homelike, comfortable, and quiet environment and an available staff of alcoholism counselors to succor the client. Medical personnel and drugs are not used. The staff helps lessen the physical effects of alcohol withdrawal by talking with clients and allaying their fears. These programs do not admit alcoholics who require medical care or have a history of severe withdrawal reactions, such as multiple seizures or delirium tremens.

The alcoholic rests for the first seventy-two hours, the most dangerous period. Severe withdrawal symptoms may occur during these first three days. (Although there have been reports of withdrawal symptoms occurring as long as four months or more after the start of detoxification, such cases are uncommon.) The trained counseling staff systematically observes the clients so that any individual who requires medical care can be referred promptly to a physician.[67]

In addition to ensuring a safe detoxification, the staff assesses a client and develops a referral plan for the continuation of treatment. During the five- to seven-day stay the staff meets with the client professionally in individual and group counseling sessions as well as alcoholism education seminars, speaks informally with the client in the dining area and lounge, and encourages the client to accept referral.

The relative advantages and disadvantages of the two treatment models are not clear. Accordingly, the Vera Institute of Justice is conducting comparison studies of three detoxification units in New York City—two targeted to the homeless and the third to the general population, including some homeless—to determine whether medical detoxification is more effective than the nonmedical model in achieving its goals.[71]

Continuing in Treatment

Although public inebriates will readily enter a five-day detoxification unit to withdraw from alcohol, they are not as successful in remaining sober and continuing in treatment after detoxification. For skid row alcoholics, the recovery period in a detoxification unit is not long enough to ensure sobriety. They must enroll in long-term treatment programs to achieve this goal. Although the detoxified individual has passed a critical state and withdrawal symptoms are not likely, alcohol effects still cloud judgment for about six months.

Certainly, a short stay in detoxification is not long enough to reorganize a life. When these people leave the detoxification unit, they have little hope of improving their environment. A number of authors in the field have noted that skid row does not provide the nourishment for sober functioning and perpetuates the use of alcohol[72] by decreasing motivation to continue treatment.

The alcoholic perceives himself as hopeless, and continuing treatment after detoxification seems futile. Many continue to deny their alcoholism, do not accept the need for lengthy treatment, and present themselves for help only when they are physically incapable of continuing the drinking episode.

The Manhattan Bowery Corporation has found that referrals are more likely to be successful when admission to a treatment program occurs on the day of discharge from the detoxification unit. Accordingly, if a preadmission interview is required, it should be done during the detoxification stay. The use of waiting lists to test the patient's motivation and potential for sobriety before offering treatment has been found inappropriate.

> The motivation concept as frequently applied to alcoholics serves as a convenient rationale for unwillingness to review and modify

current policies so as to encourage the alcoholic to seek treatment
and stay with it.[73]

Moreover, MBC's experience indicates that the use of disulfuram (Antabuse®) is a necessary adjunct for the skid row alcoholic to continue in treatment.[74]

Recommended Treatment Services

Treatment services vary in length and intensity from outpatient services to long-term institutionalization.

—Inpatient rehabilitation units are short-term (twenty-one days to eight weeks), intense, residential treatment programs. The emphasis is on helping alcoholics understand their disease in a protected treatment setting that is usually isolated from the community.

—Missions, such as the Salvation Army and the Volunteers of America, focus on the return of people to normal living schedules, helping them to acquire, regain, or upgrade work skills. Counseling and other treatment is not emphasized. These programs have flexible lengths of stay in their residential facilities that can be adapted to the needs of the patient.

—Outpatient programs provide alcoholism treatment for individuals who reside in the community or use a shelter system. They offer a range of services, including individual and group counseling, vocational assessment and rehabilitation, medical and psychiatric consultations, alcoholism education, recreational therapy, and Alcoholics Anonymous (AA) meetings. Unlike residential programs, treatment at an outpatient clinic does not have a definite time limit.[75] The time required to complete the program is determined by the progress of the patient.

—Custodial care facilities are long-term institutions that provide custodial care for individuals who are not capable of living independently.

—Halfway houses offer structured transitional residential treatment. The focus is on helping alcoholics develop vocational plans so they can become functioning members of the community. Halfway houses provide twenty-four hour supervision.

—Community residences provide alcoholics with a sober, community-living experience for six months to one year while they receive treatment at an affiliated outpatient clinic.[76,77] A community residence does not offer twenty-four hour structure and supervision, and the level of care is less comprehensive than that of a halfway house. The community residence places emphasis on independence and self-reliance; thus the residents shop for and prepare their own meals, do their own laundry, are responsible for maintenance of the residence, and govern themselves.

The distinction drawn between the halfway house and the community residence is somewhat artificial. It pertains in states such as New York where law and regulations set different standards that often determine third-party reimbursement rates. However, in states that do not mandate the distinction, the terms refer to entities that are indistinguishable.

Sequence of Treatment

Continuity of care is essential to the recovery of the homeless alcoholic. The ideal sequence of treatment is one in which alcoholics move from a structured institution, where sobriety is imposed on them, to the community, where they become independent and responsible for maintaining their sobriety.

A five- to seven-day detoxification is the first step in the treatment/ recovery process. In most cases the next step should be placement in an inpatient rehabilitation unit for one to three months. These intensive, highly structured treatment programs provide group and individual counseling, alcoholism education, psychiatric consultations, vocational and educational assessments, and Alcoholics Anonymous (AA) meetings.[78] The next referral should be to a community-based residence or halfway house for six months to a year. While residing in a therapeutic setting and receiving alcoholism treatment at an outpatient clinic, the alcoholic begins to work or to attend school and to adjust to a more regular existence. Living with other recovering alcoholics offers these people the opportunity to address problems connected with their alcoholism. These may include concern with interpersonal relationships, excessive guilt over past behavior, or difficulties at work or school. They can also develop relationships with other recovering alcoholics in AA so that a sober support system will be available when they leave the protected environment of the halfway house.

Patients continue outpatient care until discharged. At this stage, they can participate in weekly counseling sessions or a more intensive regimen, depending on need and level of deterioration.

Although this treatment sequence is desirable, all too often adherence is difficult, because the number of patient and residential beds is limited. Therefore, many patients must be referred directly to outpatient clinics.

Relapse

But what about the alcoholics who relapse? Where do they fit into the scheme? This is an important issue in the treatment of public inebriates, who relapse more frequently than other recovering alcoholics.

> In sum the composite picture of the alcoholic outpatient who is most likely to drop out of treatment is that of a field dependent, counterdependent, highly symptomatic, socially isolated lower-class person of poor social stability who is highly ambivalent about treatment and has psychopathic features. The skid row alcoholic is the most extreme example of this kind of patient.[79]

Often the skid row alcoholic does not accept referral for further treatment and relapses within hours of discharge from a detoxification unit.

> An alcoholic may be admitted to a hospital, "dried out" so physical dependence is nullified; given tranquilizers to ease withdrawal effects and subsequent nervousness; physically restored with food, exercise and vitamins; and psychologically supported through talks with a therapist and group encounter sessions. Yet, he returns to heavy drinking shortly after discharge.[80]

Workers in the detoxification facility may confront the same deteriorating alcoholics every month or even more frequently, depending on the agency's admission regulations. Clearly, the services provided in detoxification do not always help motivate individuals toward further treatment.

For many public inebriates, alcoholism treatment is a part of their drinking cycle. It has been argued that the therapeutic revolving door appears to have replaced arrest and jail.[82,83] The skid row alcoholic often uses rehabilitative agencies as survival resources for food, shelter, and clothing rather than for treatment.[84]

In 1982 the Manhattan Bowery Corporation developed a five-bed extended-stay unit that attempts to deal with the problem of easing the transition between detoxification and after-care. Based on the premise that five days in detoxification is not long enough for the chronically relapsing alcoholic to recover from the physical and psychological effects of drinking episodes, the unit extends the inpatient stay for an additional twenty-eight days. Patients are transferred to the extended-stay unit after completion of detoxification and participate in individual and group counseling, alcoholism education sessions, recreational activities, and a limited on-site work program. Also, during this time they are given assistance in obtaining financial entitlements, receive medical follow-up care, and are encouraged to accept the need for continued long-term care. Data collected on the unit indicate the program has been successful in achieving its goal. Eighty-eight percent of those who completed the program became involved in outpatient treatment after discharge from the extended-stay program,[80] compared to 33 percent of those who were treated only in the MBC's detoxification units. A substantial number of those who completed the program have maintained periods of sobriety for up to seven months.[81]

SUMMARY

Despite the frequency of relapses and the underlying motives the homeless alcoholic might have for entering a rehabilitative unit, treatment can have a major impact on the health and well-being of public inebriates. A significant number do recover and maintain long-term sobriety. Many others are sober for substantial periods of time between drinking bouts. These periods of sobriety mean improved physical and mental health and greater social stability.

We now know that damage to the liver and other organs is often arrested and reversed in the recovery process. Even some brain damage is reversible. Interruptions of the drinking cycle allow skid row alcoholics to maintain rooms in single-room-occupancy hotels, hold jobs, maintain affiliations with AA, continue medical treatment for chronic problems, and develop and retain friendships. Although such people may have as many as three or four relapses per year, they are able to function at a much higher level after their introduction to treatment.

Skid row alcoholics have a rate of recovery from alcoholism that is far lower than that of the general population, yet they, like their middle-class counterparts, suffer from a disease that can be arrested with treatment. Proper treatment for the public inebriate involves a variety of therapeutic interventions used over an extended period of time. Success is possible and should be sought.

REFERENCES

1. Report of the board of trustees of the AMA. JAMA. 1956; 162:749.
2. Powell v. Texas, 392 U.S. 514 (1968).
3. Nimmer RT. Two million unnecessary arrests. American Bar Foundation, 1971:1-5.
4. Murtagh JM. Arrests for public intoxication. Fordham Law Review. 1966; 35(1):1-14.
5. Comprehensive Alcohol Abuse and Alcohol Prevention, Treatment and Rehabilitation Act of 1970, P.L. 91-616 84 Stat. 1848 (1970).
6. U.S., Department of Health, Education and Welfare, NIAAA 1972a, Alcoholic and alcoholism, problems, programs and progress, no. 72-9127. Public Law 91-616 S-38835, 1970.
7. U.S., Department of Health, Education and Welfare. The role of the law in improving the quality of life of the public inebriates: Proceedings of seminar on public health services and the public inebriate, prepared by Manos SS, no. (ADM) 75-218, 1975:20-32.
8. Notes on a visit to St. Louis Detox Program, Manhattan Bowery Corporation, 1967 (unpublished).
9. In lieu of arrest: the Manhattan Bowery Project treatment for homeless alcoholics. New York: The Criminal Justice Coordinating Council of New York City and Vera Institute of Justice, 1969.
10. Ten-year report of the Manhattan Bowery Corporation: 1967 to 1977. New York: Manhattan Bowery Corporation, 1977.
11. Further work in criminal justice reform. New York: Vera Institute of Justice, 1977:41-44.
12. P.L. 94-371; 90 State. 1035 (1976); 42 U.S.C. 4551 et seq.
13. Finister D. A history of public inebriate programs in the United States. Rockville, Maryland: National Institute of Alcohol Abuse and Alcoholism, 1984.
14. Todd MC. How future physicians must see the alcoholic. Rhode Island Med J. 1975; 75:389-401.
15. Manual on Alcoholism. 3rd edition. Chicago: American Medical Association, 1977.
16. Seixas FA. Criteria for the diagnosis of alcoholism. In: Estes NJ, Heinemann ME, eds. Alcoholism: development, consequences and interventions, 2nd edition. St. Louis: C. V. Mosby, 1982:49-67.
17. U.S., Department of Health and Human Services, National directory of drug abuse and alcoholism treatment programs, no. (ADM) 83-321, 1983.
18. Personal Communication. National Coalition on Jail Reform. Washington DC, NIAAA Clearinghouse, June 1984.
19. Geffner EI. Proceedings of conference on public inebriate policy, California state department of alcohol and drug programs. New York: Manhattan Bowery Corporation, 1980.
20. Proceedings of conference on public inebriates: overview and alternatives to jail. Milwaukee, The National Coalition for Jail Reform, June 1983.

21. Aaronson DE, Dienes DT, Musheno MC. Improving police discretion rationality in handling public inebriates (Parts I & II). Administrative Law Review, American Bar Association, 29(4), 1977; 30(1), 1978.
22. Blume SB. The public inebriate and public policy: an outline for discussion. Presented at a meeting of NIAAA on public inebriate issues. Chevy Chase, MD., April 1981.
23. Kissin B. Theory and practice in the treatment of alcoholism. In: Kissin B, Begleiter H, eds. The biology of alcoholism. Vol. 5. New York, Plenum Press, 1977:1–51.
24. Ten Leading Causes of Death. National Center for Health Statistics, 1982.
25. Kissin B. Medical management of the alcoholic patient. In: Kissin B, Begleiter H, eds. The biology of alcoholism. Vol. 5. New York: Plenum Press, 1977:53–103.
26. Zimberg S. Alcoholism prevalence in emergency rooms and walk-in clinics. NYS J Med. 1979; 9:1533–36.
27. Dorland's illustrated medical dictionary. 26th edition. Philadelphia, W. B. Saunders, 1981:45.
28. Selzer ML. Alcoholism and alcoholic psychoses. In: Kaplin HI, Freedman AM, Sadock BJ, eds. Comprehensive textbook of psychiatry. 3rd edition. Vol. 2. Baltimore: Williams and Wilkins, 1980:1629–45.
29. Murray RM, Stabnau JR. Genetic factors in alcoholism predisposition. In: Pattison EM and Kaufmann E, eds. Encyclopedic handbook of alcoholism. New York: Gardner Press, 1982:135–44.
30. Jellinek EM. Phases of alcohol addiction. Q J Stud Alcohol. 1952; 13:673–84.
31. Pittman DJ, Gordon CW. Revolving door: a study of the chronic police case inebriate. Glencoe, Illinois: The Free Press, 1958.
32. Bahr HM, Garret GR. Women alone: the disaffiliation of urban females. Lexington, Mass.: Heath, 1978.
33. Bogue DJ. Skid row in American cities. Chicago: University of Chicago Press, 1963.
34. Bahr HM, Caplow T. Old men drunk and sober. New York: University Press, 1973.
35. Cahalon D, Cisin IH, Crossley HM. American drinking practices: a national study of drinking behavior and attitudes. New Brunswick N.J.: Rutgers Center for Alcohol Studies, Monograph No. 6, 1969.
36. Hopper K, Baxter E. One year later. New York: Community Services Society, 1982.
37. Crystal S. Chronic and situational dependency: long-term residents in a shelter for men. New York: Human Resources Administration, Family and Adult Services, May 1982.
38. Crystal S. New arrivals: first-time shelter clients. New York: Human Resources Administration, Family and Adult Services, November 1982.
39. Bellamy C. From country asylums to city streets: the contradiction between deinstitutionalization and state mental health funding priorities. New York: The City of New York Council, June 1979.
40. Five-year plan for alcoholism services: New York City, 1984–1988. New

York: NYC Dept of Mental Health, Mental Retardation and Alcoholism Services, July 1983.

41. New York State Psychiatric Institute. Evaluation of Goddard-Riverside project reach-out. New York: Community Evaluation Program of NYS Psychiatric Institute, 1981–82.
42. Community support system preliminary report. New York: CSS Evaluation Program, Psychiatric Institute, 1983.
43. Smith-DiJulio K, Heinemann ME, Busch L. Care of the alcoholic patient during acute episodes. In: Estes NJ, Heinemann ME, eds. Alcoholism: development, consequences and intervention. 2nd Edition. St. Louis, C. V. Mosby, 1982:270–82.
44. Kurtz NR, Googins R, Hovard WC. Measuring the success of occupational alcoholism programs. J Stud Alcohol. 1984; 45(1):33–45.
45. Rubington E. The role of the halfway house in the rehabilitation of alcoholics. In: Kissin B, Begleiter H, eds. The biology of alcoholism. Vol. 5. New York: Plenum Press, 1977:351–83.
46. Kiernan E. Residential treatment—a model treating alcoholics who are disaffiliated: Manhattan Bowery Project's STEP I. Tel Aviv, Proceedings of 2nd International Congress on Drugs and Alcohol, 1983.
47. Case Records: Psychosocial and Medical Histories. New York: Manhattan Bowery Corporation, 1967–1984.
48. Thompson AD. There may yet be time to save your brain (editorial). Brit J Alcohol & Alcoholism. 1980; 15(3):89–92.
49. Bergenan H, Borg S, Hindmarsh T. Computerized tomography of the brain and neuropsychiatric assessment of male alcoholic patients and a random sample of the general population. Acta Psych Scand (suppl.). 1980; 286:77–88.
50. Carlen PL, Wilkenson DA. Alcoholic brain damage and reversible defects. Acta Psych Scand (suppl.). 1980; 286:103–18.
51. Parson OA. Brain damage in alcoholics: altered states of unconsciousness. In: Gross MM, ed. Alcohol intoxication and withdrawal: experimental studies II. New York: Plenum Press, 1975:569–84.
52. Victor M, Adams RD. Deficiency diseases of the nervous system. In: Petersdorf et al., eds. Harrison's principles of internal medicine. 10th edition. Vol. 2. New York: McGraw-Hill, 1983:2112–18.
53. Behse F, Buchthal F. Alcoholic neuropathy: clinical electrophysiologic and biopsy finding. Ann Neurol. 1976; 26:368.
54. Feinman L. Treatment of bleeding in the alcoholic. Practical Gastroenterology. 1983; 6(3):18–25.
55. Mezey E. Gastrointestinal complication of alcoholism. Practical Gastroenterology. 1983; 6(3):7–17.
56. Palmer ED. Gastritis: a re-evaluation. Medicine. 1954; 33:199–290.
57. Krasner B, Thompson T. Gastric epithelial cell turnover after acute and chronic alcohol ingestion. Grit. 1974; 15:336.
58. Burnett DA, Sorrell MF. Alcoholic cirrhosis in alcohol and the GI tract. Clinics in Gastroenterology. 1981; 10(2):443–56.

59. Leevy CM. Clinical diagnosis, evaluation and treatment of liver disease in alcoholics. Fed Proc. 1967; 26:1474–81.
60. Lieber CS. Metabolic effects of ethanol on the liver and other digestive organs. Clinics in Gastroenterology. 1981; 10(2):315–42.
61. Powell WJ, Klatskin G. Duration of survival in patients with Laennec's cirrhosis. Am J Med. 1967; 44:406–20.
62. Maxwell DS. Developmental effects of alcohol. Ann Intern Med. 1984; 100:405–16.
63. Regan TJ, Ettinger PO, Tyons MM, et al. Ethyl alcohol as a cardiac risk factor. Current Problems in Cardiology. 1977; 2:1–35.
64. Klatsky AL. Alcohol and cardiovascular disorders. Primary Cardiology. 1979; 10:76–83.
65. Glatt MM. Group therapy in alcoholism treatment. Brit J Addiction. 1958; 54(2):133–48.
66. Whitfield CL, Thompson G, Lamb A, et al. Detoxification of 1,024 alcoholic patients without psychoactive drugs. JAMA. 1978; 239:1409–10.
67. Sparadeo FR, Zwick WR, Ruggiero SD, et al. Evaluation of a social setting detoxification program. J Stud Alcohol. 1982; 43:1125.
68. O'Briant R, Peterson NW, Heacock D. How safe is social setting detoxification? Alcohol Health & Res World. 1977; 1(2):22–27.
69. Favozza AR. The alcohol withdrawal syndrome and medical detoxification. In: Pattison, EM, Kaufman E, eds. Encyclopedic handbook of alcoholism. New York: Gardner Press, 1982:1068–75.
70. First Annual Report, Manhattan Bowery Corporation. New York: Manhattan Bowery Corporation, 1968.
71. The impact of alcohol detoxification programs (grant proposal). New York: Vera Institute of Justice, 1982.
72. Bates M. Using the environment to help the male skid row alcoholic. Social Casework: J Contemporary Soc Work. 1983; 64(5):276–82.
73. Stern MW, Pittman E. The concept of motivation: a source of institutional and professional blockage in the treatment of alcoholics. Q J Stud Alcohol. 1965; 26:20–41.
74. Morgan RR, Cagan EJ. Acute alcohol intoxication, the disulfiram reaction, and methyl alcohol intoxication. In: Kissin B, Begleiter H, eds. The biology of alcoholism. Vol. 3. New York: Plenum Press, 1974:163–89.
75. Part 330, New York State Law Governing Operation of Alcoholism Outpatient Services, 1979.
76. Turner S. Community residential treatment for the skid row alcoholic. J Health & Soc Work. 1979; 4:163–80.
77. Dolan J, Kiernan E. A multi-program approach to alcoholism services for the public inebriate. New York: NY Academy of Sciences, 1976.
78. Wilson WG. Alcoholics anonymous: the story of how many thousands of men and women have recovered from alcoholism. 3rd edition. New York: AA World Services, 1976.
79. Baekeland F, Lundwall L. Engaging the alcoholic in treatment and keeping him there. The biology of alcoholism. 1977; 5:161–95.

80. Wiseman JP. Sober time: the neglected variables in recidivism of alcoholic persons. In: Chafetz ME, ed. Proceedings. U.S., Department of Health, Education, and Welfare, no. (NIH) 74-676, 1973.
81. Data collected on Extended Care unit at Manhattan Bowery Corporation, Jan 1982–Dec 1983.
82. Rodin MB, Pickup L, Morton DR, Keatings C. Gimme shelter: ethnographic perspectives on skid row inebriates in detoxification centers. Chicago: University of Illinois School of Public Health, 1982.
83. Sagan RW, Mauss AL. Padding the revolving door: an initial assessment of the Uniform Alcoholism and Intoxification Treatment Act. Soc Problems. 1978; 26:232–47.
84. Wiseman JP. Stations of the lost: the treatment of skid row alcoholics. Chicago: University of Chicago Press, 1979.

11

Tuberculosis: An Overview

Michael Iseman

From 1947 to 1952, when isoniazid, streptomycin, and para-amino-salicylic were discovered, tuberculosis (TB) went from a disease with a less than 50 percent five-year survival rate to merely another infectious disorder that was curable in almost every instance. In the early days of chemotherapy, patients with tuberculosis were cared for in sanitoria, where virtually every dose of medication could be assured. Long-term hospital care was provided through public funding. Patient compliance—that it, willingness to remain in the sanitorium for the duration of treatment—was enforced by the strong sway this ancient killer held over the public.

TREATMENT NONCOMPLIANCE

In the modern era of chemotherapy, tuberculosis has moved into the mainstream of medical care. TB sanitoria have closed, specialty clinics been curtailed, and long-term inpatient care abandoned in favor of ambulatory treatment. Unfortunately, these changes have resulted in a substantially worse outcome in many TB cases. As tuberculosis has receded in the public's perception as an ominous disease, both lay and professional concern has substantially diminished. By shifting chemotherapy to the outpatient setting, we have invited many patients in the best of circumstances either to abandon treatment or to take their medications so erratically that treatment failures or relapses ensue, frequently with drug-resistant organisms. Such noncompliance is now the major factor thwarting successful TB chemotherapy in America's large urban centers. In a recent U.S. Public Health Service short-course chemotherapy trial[1] in major cities across the country, roughly 26 percent of the patients left the study or broke the protocol within six months.

Noncompliance among patients is to be expected. More disheartening is noncompliance on the part of caregivers. Tuberculosis is a communicable disease and is included explicity or implicitly in public health laws and regulations in every major municipality, county, and state in our country. Public health officers are charged with enforcing these regulations. However, through lack of interest, lack of resolve, and/or inadequate resources, few governmental entities consistently attempt to enforce the statutes regarding tuberculosis.

DOUBLE JEOPARDY

We can use the term *double jeopardy* in the context of tuberculosis in the homeless to indicate two phenomena: 1) the homeless in America are at high risk of developing tuberculosis, and 2) once these individuals are afflicted with this disease, poor nutrition, crowded shelters, and their stressful lifestyle conspire to make it unlikely that they will receive curative chemotherapy.

We are at the end of an epidemiological epoch: a 500-year cycle of epidemic tuberculosis inherited from Europe has substantially receded in this century. A variety of circumstances—including Darwinian selection, improved nutrition, more hygienic housing, the sanitorium movement with patient isolation, and chemotherapy—has led to a dramatic overall reduction in the prevalence of tuberculosis in both Europe and North America. However, as this tidal wave has receded, it has left behind residual pools of infection and encapsulated mini-epidemics within confined groups in America. The most notable of these today include the elderly, minorities, recent immigrants, and substance abusers. These groups contribute substantially to the ranks of the homeless.

Data from the U.S. Public Health Service (USPHS)[2] reveal a strikingly increased risk for tuberculosis among the elderly. Since TB was still rampant in the first decades of this century, the vast majority of today's elderly were exposed to tuberculosis in childhood. Over half of the urban high school graduates at the turn of the century had a positive tuberculin skin test, evidence of tuberculosis infection. Most of these individuals, in their sixth, seventh, and eighth decades, have remained free of overt tuberculosis disease until now, when a variety of factors have combined to diminish their immunological defenses and tip the balance in favor of the mycobacterium. Among these factors surely must be numbered the stresses of inadequate housing and nutrition for many older people. USPHS 1980[2] data reveal the following prevalence rates for these age groups, expressed as cases of disease per 100,000 persons per year: Overall = 12.3; 20–34 years = 9; 35–44 years = 14; 45–54 years = 18; 55–64 years = 20; and over 65 years = 31.

Many members of minority groups have recently come from regions where tuberculosis is still epidemic. Only a small percentage arrive in the United States with active disease. A far greater number arrive in the country infected but without overt disease; subsequently, under the stresses associated with the immigrant lifestyle, they develop active tuberculosis. Extraordinarily crowded housing or transient sleeping quarters promote the spread of this infection, which under ordinary circumstances is only minimally contagious. By the practice of staying with friends or family, recent arrivals act as vectors to promote disease among established or second generation immigrant communities. Data from Colorado,[3] which are typical of national statistics, indicate strikingly disparate rates of tuberculosis among various racial or ethnic groups. Expressed as cases per 100,000 population per year they are: whites = 4, blacks = 12, whites with Spanish surnames = 15, American Indians = 75, and Southeast Asians = approximately 1,000.

Another pool of tuberculosis in America exists among substance abusers. By far the most prominent group here is the alcoholic. There is a strong association between tuberculosis and alcohol abuse. Exact data are difficult to obtain on the prevalence of TB in this group. However, estimates of tuberculosis case rates in unaffiliated or homeless urban alcoholics range as high as 500 per 100,000 per year.

Hard data are also difficult to obtain for TB case rates among the other large group of substance abusers, heroin addicts. Nevertheless, limited surveys indicate a high level of both tuberculosis infection and disease among this group of patients.

REFERENCES

1. Snider, DE, Long MW, Cross, S, Farer L. Six months Isoniazid-Rifampin therapy for pulmonary tuberculosis: report of a United States Public Health Service cooperative trial. Am Rev Resp Dis. 1984; 129:573–79.
2. U.S., Department of Health and Human Services, Center for Disease Control. Tuberculosis statistics: states and cities, 1980, no. (CDC) 82-8249.
3. Colorado Dept of Health. Colorado Disease Bulletin 7: Issue 36, Sept 1979.

12

Tuberculosis in the SRO/Homeless Population

John McAdam, Philip W. Brickner,
Roslynn Glicksman, Dearborn Edwards,
Brian Fallon, and Philip Yanowitch

New York City's case and death rates for pulmonary tuberculosis have fallen dramatically since the advent of public health measures and antibiotic therapy, but there remains a persistent focus of infection.[1-3] For those living on our streets, in our shelters, and in our single-room-occupancy (SRO) hotels, tuberculosis—the white plague of the nineteenth century—is a constant companion.

In the 1970s, a trend was noted among tuberculosis patients admitted to St. Vincent's Hospital in New York City: many were found to be residents of SRO hotels on Manhattan's lower West Side. A study by Sherman and others was undertaken to determine the scope of the problem.[4] Two-hundred-fifty individuals living in three SROs were chosen for evaluation of their PPD (Purified Protein Derivative) skin test status. (See Figure 12.1.) Of these, 191 accepted skin testing; 0.1

The work reported herein was assisted by a generous grant from the Gateposts Foundation. The New York City Department of Health, Bureau of Tuberculosis, provided bacteriologic services, supplied antituberculous medications and supported summer fellows. The Human Resources Administration, New York City, provided contractual support for this work in various shelters. St. Vincent's Hospital and Medical Center of New York gave staff, administrative, radiology and ancillary support.

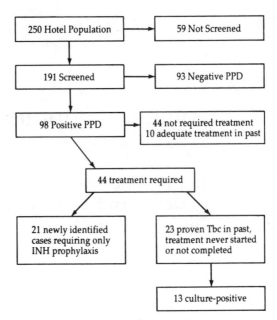

Figure 12.1. PPD Skin Test Status of SRO Residents (From Sherman MN, Brickner PW, Schwartz MS, et al. Tuberculosis in single-room-occupancy hotel residents: a persisting focus of disease. NY Med Quart. Fall 1980, p. 40. Copyright © by New York Medical College, 1980. Reprinted with permission.)

cc of Tween-stabilized, intermediate strength 5TU of PPD was injected intradermally for this purpose. Ninety-eight (51 percent) of those tested were PPD-positive, indicating at least a dormant tuberculosis infection.

Ten PPD-positive participants had been appropriately treated in the past for either active or dormant tuberculosis infection. Forty-four did not meet the American Thoracic Society's suggested criteria for initiation of treatment.[5] Another forty-four, however, did meet these criteria. Of these, twenty-one required chemoprophylaxis, and twenty-three had proven untreated or inadequately treated tuberculous disease from the past. Of these twenty-three individuals, thirteen had sputum cultures positive for Mycobacterium tuberculosis. In other words, 6.7 percent of the population tested had active tuberculosis.

This preliminary analysis also evaluated PPD reactor rates according to sex, age, and race. (See Table 12.1.) Of the 191 persons studied, nineteen were women, and of these, three were PPD-positive. One hundred seventy-two subjects were men, and ninety-five, or 55 percent, were PPD-positive. Significantly, the PPD reactor rate increased from 20 percent in the third decade of life to a 73 percent peak in the seventh decade. Although the PPD reactor rate is known to increase with age in the United States, the percentage of PPD-positive reactors in the general population does not approach the high rates obtained through this study.

In 1980, an estimated 2 to 5 percent of young adults in the United States were PPD-positive, while 15 percent of those older than fifty years were positive.[6] Our figures for SRO residents were about four times as high. One possible explanation is that the increased PPD reactor rate with age was more a function of the length of time people had lived in an SRO than of absolute age. This question could not be answered in Sherman's early study.

Certain problems were evident. Of the thirteen residents with cul-

Table 12.1. Reactor Rate According to Sex, Race, and Age

		PPD Reactors	
Subject	*Total #*	*#*	*%*
Sex			
Male	172	95	55
Female	19	3	16
Total	191	98	51
Race			
White	95	43	45
Black	78	45	58
Hispanic	18	10	56
Total	191	98	51
Age			
20–29	15	3	20
30–39	35	13	37
40–49	52	27	52
50–59	43	28	65
60–69	26	19	73
70–79	6	2	33
Age Unknown	14	6	43
Total	191	98	Ave. 51

(From Sherman MN, Brickner PW, Schwartz MS, et al. Tuberculosis in single-room-occupancy hotel residents: a persisting focus of disease. NY Med Quart. Fall 1980, p. 40. Copyright © by New York Medical College, 1980. Reprinted with permission.)

ture-positive tuberculosis, ten, or 77 percent refused further treatment. Only three patients complied with a standard treatment regimen. Of the 191 subjects tested, only 166 could be ranked according to the American Thoracic Society classification. Twenty-five individuals with PPD-intermediate-positive skin tests refused chest x-rays.

Tuberculosis therapy can be an arduous process, requiring many months, or even years, of compliance in taking medication. Residents of SRO hotels tend to be individuals who cannot easily negotiate the frustrations and complexity of a hospital's typical outpatient department but are not able to afford the service of a private physician. These individuals form a medically underserved population, regardless of their geographic proximity to traditional health care systems.

Patients' compliance with antituberculosis therapy can be affected by the attitude of health care personnel. Crocco and associates[7] had fair success in treating alcoholic patients with tuberculosis. They interviewed patients who were undergoing "disciplinary discharge" following multiple episodes of drunkenness, abusive behavior, or fighting with other patients and hospital staff at Kings County Hospital in Brooklyn, where they were being treated for active tuberculosis. They stressed to patients that their doctors were personally interested in their problems, that a cure was absolutely dependent on taking medication, that alcoholism is a disease and not a moral depravity, and that patients would be welcomed in the clinic, even if intoxicated. Sixty-three percent (34 patients) completed therapy.

PRESENT STUDY

In 1980, about the time Sherman's work was published,[4] St. Vincent's Hospital's Department of Community Medicine became involved in a major expansion of its existing medical outreach programs. Teams of nurses, physicians, and social workers brought medical care to more SROs. Patients could also attend a primary care clinic at the hospital, where they received medical care from the same team members who visited them in the SROs. At this clinic, patients had access to expanded services, such as laboratory, radiology, and subspecialty clinics. In this way trust was established and a more secure therapeutic bond formed between patients and members of the medical team.

At the same time, the outreach teams also began to serve more shelters in New York City. The matter of tuberculosis soon surfaced again. Several individuals were found to be severely ill, unable to get out of bed. They were found to be suffering from disseminated tuberculosis. In a few cases, this was only discovered at autopsy.

At times it seems the homeless and SRO populations live in the preantibiotic era because of the difficulties they have in negotiating our complex health care system. Because tuberculosis is a chronic disease and may cause few or no symptoms for decades, it is especially difficult to elicit compliance with treatment regimens in this population. They have to be convinced in concrete terms that the medical team is trying to help them, as the following example from our own experience shows.

C. W. is a fifty-five year old man, resident in a New York City shelter and a heavy alcohol user at times. He first became known to our medical team in 1982 when he appeared with prescriptions for isoniazid and rifampin given to him following a recent hospitalization. His prescriptions were filled and he was given a one-month supply of medications with instructions for follow-up. C. W. soon went on a drinking binge and was lost to follow-up. Several months later he appeared again at our clinic door with more prescriptions for antituberculous medications. In the interval he had been readmitted to the hospital with active tuberculosis. Once more, the staff at the clinic sat down with him and tried to explain the importance of his medication: that it might save his life. He again promised to take his medication and to follow through with his visits to us.

In spite of our efforts, he disappeared a second time, only to show up several weeks later, now with prescriptions for three antituberculous medications, isoniazid, Rifampin©, and ethambutol. Cavitary tuberculosis, a more severe form of the disease, had developed.

The clinic staff spent more time with C. W., and an interesting fact came to light: his reactivations of tuberculosis coincided with his drinking binges. He had not stopped taking his medications because he had lost or forgotten them, but because he had been told by a well-meaning hospital physician that he could not drink alcohol and take his medication at the same time. There was concern about possible development of liver disease caused by the combined effects of isonazid and alcohol on the liver. C. W. actually had more trust in this physician's advice than most patients. He was not going to take the chance of developing side effects with our medications by combining them with alcohol. He simply stopped treatment.

This information was taken to heart by the medical staff. One shelter nurse in particular developed an especially strong therapeutic relationship with C. W. He now had a bed assigned in the shelter near her medical clinic and received his antituberculous medications daily from the medical staff. He was told that if he was drinking, he could still come for his medicine, and that the staff would tolerate anything but abusive behavior. Liver function tests were performed regularly. C. W. knows that the staff is there to help him, and that they care about him as an individual. He also knows that if he forgets to come for his medication one of us will go looking for him to remind him.

The result is that C. W. has completed eleven months of continuous antituberculous therapy. He has gained weight and no longer has night sweats or a productive cough. His sputum has been negative for tuberculi bacilli for the past eight months. He is well on his way toward completion of an eighteen- to twenty-four-month regimen for a cure.

CHALLENGE

Since we know that active cases of tuberculosis are common in this population, we began to suspect a high prevalence of dormant tuberculous infection as well. Trying to detect this disease process in the homeless population is a challenge. The diagnosis of tuberculous infection requires more than one clinic visit. An already suspicious individual must be convinced that he or she should let the doctor or nurse give an intradermal injection, a PPD skin test, just to find a disease that is not causing any discomfort. The patient also must be motivated to return to have the skin test read, with the possibility of having to submit to a physical examination, blood tests, sputum collection, and a chest x-ray. All of this must be done before initiation of prophylactic therapy that may require a year or more of daily medication. Homeless people are much more likely to be concerned with obtaining food or shelter for the night. A medical team's success in guiding a patient through this maze of evaluation and follow-up can be a real measure of the client's trust in its members.[3]

After experiences with patients like C. W., the staff began to suspect that tuberculosis was a major health problem in the SRO/Homeless population. We decided to undertake a study of sufficient size to provide significant data regarding the magnitude of this issue in our patients. Towards this end, we have begun an analysis that will ultimately incorporate data on about 5000 homeless persons.

People enter the tuberculosis study voluntarily. Selection is not random. Common reasons for participation include tuberculosis screening as a prerequisite for job training and placement; appearance at a shelter clinic because of intercurrent illness; individual desire to have tuberculosis ruled out; or fear because a companion or roommate has developed the illness.

Staff members use a standard questionnaire. If a past history of a positive tuberculosis skin test is obtained, further questions are asked in order to determine whether the patient is a candidate for either prophylactic treatment or therapy for active tuberculosis, following the criteria of the American Thoracic Society and the Centers for Disease Control.[7,8] If there is no prior history of a positive skin test, patients are given Tween-stabilized Purified Protein Derivative (PPD) 5 TU and Candida extract 1:1000 0.1 cc intradermally. The latter is used to insure that a negative PPD is truly negative, not falsely negative due to anergy.

PPD skin test results fall into the following categories:

- Negative (<5 mm of skin induration at 48 hours)
- Intermediate (5 to 10 mm)
- Positive (>10 mm)
- Positive by history

Anergy tests are considered positive when >5 mm of erythema are present at the injection site in twenty-four to forty-eight hours. If there is a negative test with candida extract, a second injection of a different antigen, trichophyton 1:100 extract, is used. If the individual still does not react, then an evaluation is started to rule out diseases that blunt the normal delayed hypersensitivity reaction. When patients present with evident active pulmonary tuberculosis, skin tests are not used.

People with positive skin tests are offered chest x-rays. Following this, if indicated, sputum cultures are obtained. For those who demonstrate evidence of active disease, a standard antituberculous treatment regimen is instituted. For those whose disease is deemed dormant, a prophylactic regimen is offered, using isoniazid therapy. This is a well-documented and effective method of preventing reactivation of dormant tuberculosis.[8,9] All patients who receive antituberculous therapy are followed closely by the health care team for evidence of drug toxicity, a recognized hazard of this form of treatment.[8]

RESULTS

To date, our study includes 729 individuals, comprised of 661 SRO and shelter residents and 68 staff members of three shelters. Basic demographic data for those in the study, concerning race, sex, mean educational level, and mean age are demonstrated in Tables 12.2 and 12.3. The population is predominantly male and white in the SROs; male and black in the shelters. The SRO group is older. Overall, PPD reactor rates

Table 12.2. Demographic Data by Site: Hotels (n = 129) (Saint Vincent's Hospital Department of Community Medicine Tuberculosis Study, September 1982–June 1984)

	Woodstock		Jane West		Keller	
Race						
Unknown	0		1	2%	1	2%
White	18	72%	25	42%	21	47%
Black	2	8%	25	42%	20	44%
Asian	4	16%	0		0	
Hispanic	1	4%	8	14%	3	7%
Other	0		0		0	
Total	25	100%	59	100%	45	100%
Sex						
Male	18	72%	54	92%	41	91%
Female	7	28%	5	8%	4	9%
Total	25	100%	59	100%	45	100%
Education						
Mean # Yrs.	10		10		10	
Age						
Mean # Yrs.	70		51		45	

were higher for SRO residents (51 percent) than for those in shelters (41 percent). In contrast, the majority of active tuberculosis cases (26 of the 30 cases) were found at shelters, particularly at the Keener building shelter on Ward's Island.

Active Tuberculosis

The active tuberculosis cases represent 4.3 percent of all those persons in the study to date and 8.5% of those studied at the Keener building. Our best estimate is that thus far about 15 to 20 percent of all residents in the shelters have been incorporated into the study. Because selection is not random, these figures may change significantly as a larger fraction of the total population is evaluated.

On any given day, the Keener building on Ward's Island gives shelter to over 800 homeless men. It is also a major center of active tuberculosis. (See Table 12.4.) Twenty-six people with or under treatment for the active disease are known to have lived, slept, and eaten at the shelter during the time of the study. One can only guess at the number of unknown cases. Our data permit a specific analysis of the known cases with respect to the clients' age, race, level of alcohol consumption, and classification as cases of "new" or "old" tuberculosis.

Clients being treated for active tuberculosis (see Table 12.5) had a mean age of 38.6 years, a figure not differing significantly from the mean age of 36.0 years found for the study population as a whole. The group's median age was 32.5 years; in other words, half of those being treated for the active disease were under 33 years of age. This is indeed a very young group. Of those with "new" (to be defined below) cases of the active disease, the mean age was 37.0 and the median age 32 years.

The racial composition of the group with active tuberculosis (both "new" and "old" cases) is similar to that of the study population as a whole. Of the individuals in the latter group whose racial backgrounds are known, 68% (173 out of 253) were black. Of those with active tuberculosis, the comparable figure is 72% (18 out of 25). Both groups had

Table 12.3. Demographic Data by Site: Shelters (n = 532) (Saint Vincent's Hospital Department of Community Medicine Tuberculosis Study, September 1982–June 1984)

	Keener Building		Manhattan Bowery		Men's Shelter		Moravian Church		Westside Cluster	
Race										
Unknown	52	17%	0		9	34%	4	5%	2	4%
White	47	16%	33	41%	3	11%	49	65%	20	47%
Black	173	57%	30	38%	12	44%	20	27%	17	40%
Hispanic	33	10%	16	20%	2	7%	2	3%	3	7%
Asian	0		1	1%	0		0		0	
Other	2		0		1	4%	0		1	2%
Total	307	100%	80	100%	27	100%	75	100%	43	100%
Sex										
Unknown	0		0		0		3	4%	0	
Male	307		80		27		34	45%	0	
Female	0		0		0		38	51%	43	
Total	307		80		27		75	100%	43	
Education										
Mean # Yrs.	11.2		NK		NK		12.0		11.7	
Age										
Mean # Yrs.	35.8		42.3		36.1		47.5		45.0	

Total Individuals Screened = 661 Client + 68 Staff = 729

Table 12.4.   PPD Reactor Rate by Site: Hotels (n = 129); Shelters (n = 529) (Saint Vincent's Hospital Department of Community Medicine Tuberculosis Study, September 1982–June 1984)*

	Woodstock		Jane West		Keller	
Negative	16	64%	28	48%	18	40%
Intermediate	0		0		1	2%
Positive	9	36%	25	42%	23	51%
Positive by hx	0		4	7%	2	5%
Active Tb	0		2	3%	1	2%
Total	25	100%	59	100%	45	100%

	Keener Building		Men's Shelter		Manhattan Bowery		Moravian Church		Westside Cluster	
Negative	161	53%	16	59%	41	51%	50	67%	32	74%
Intermediate	7	2%	2	7%	1	1%	0		2	5%
Positive	99	33%	8	30%	32	40%	23	30%	9	21%
Positive by hx	11	4%	0		6	8%	2	3%	0	
Active Tb	26	8.5%	1	4%	0		0		0	
Total	304	100.5%	27	100%	80	100%	75	100%	43	100%

*Percentages that do not total 100 do so due to rounding.

lesser numbers of whites and Hispanics. There were no Asians in the study population.

With respect to drinking habits, we have adequate data for 17 of the 26 people treated for the active disease. Based on interviews, we classified only 5 of the 17 as heavy drinkers or former heavy drinkers (see the definitions accompanying Table 12.6). This finding contests the notion that active tuberculosis at the shelters is a problem limited predominantly to noncompliant alcoholics.

We define a "new" case of tuberculosis as one in which the patient received a first-time diagnosis of active tuberculosis during the period of the study, or else had been taking medication for such a case, without interruption of more than one month, for a time period extending into that of the study. These individuals with new, active tuberculosis are classified in Table 12.5 according to whether or not they were living at Keener when the diagnosis was made.

"Old" cases of tuberculosis (Table 12.5)—those active at Keener at some point in the study period, yet not meeting the criteria for new cases—represent individuals for whom previous therapy had failed, presumably because of noncompliance with the treatment regimen. We determined that cases were old by cross-checking the histories we ob-

Table 12.5. Active Tuberculosis Cases at the Keener Building Shelter (Saint Vincent's Hospital Department of Community Medicine Tuberculosis Study, September 1982–June 1984)

	Study Population	Total Active TB Cases	New TB Cases	New TB Cases Diagnosed While Client Lived at Keener	New TB Cases Diagnosed While Client Lived Elsewhere than Keener	Old TB Cases Active at Keener
Race						
White	47 (15%)	4 (15%)	3 (14%)	1 (9%)	2 (20%)	1 (20%)
Hispanic	33 (11%)	3 (12%)	3 (14%)	2 (18%)	1 (10%)	0 (0%)
Black	173 (56%)	18 (69%)	14 (67%)	8 (73%)	6 (60%)	4 (80%)
Unknown	52 (17%)	1 (4%)	1 (5%)	0 (0%)	1 (10%)	0 (0%)
Other	2 (1%)	0 (0%)	0 (0%)	0 (0%)	0 (0%)	0 (0%)
Total	307 (100%)	26 (100%)	21 (100%)	11 (100%)	10 (100%)	5 (100%)
Mean age	36.0 (n = 235)	38.6 (n = 26)	37 (n = 21)	36.3 (n = 11)	37.7 (n = 10)	45.6
Median age		32.5 (n = 26)	32 (n = 21)	31 (n = 11)	32 (n = 10)	48
Heavy drinkers (present and former)	90 (38%) (n = 236)	5 (29%) (n = 17)	2 (15%) (n = 13)	0 (0%) (n = 7)	2 (33%) (n = 6)	3 (15%) (n = 4)

Category	% of Study Population
Total active TB cases	8.5%
New TB cases	6.8%
New TB cases diagnosed while client resided at Keener	3.6%
New TB cases diagnosed while client resided elsewhere than Keener	3.2%
Old TB cases active at Keener	1.6%

Table 12.6.   PPD Reactor Rate vs. Alcohol Use (n = 497) (Saint Vincent's Hospital Department of Community Medicine Tuberculosis Study, September 1982–June 1984)

	Heavy Drinkers		Former Drinkers		Light Drinkers		Nondrinkers	
Negative	64	48%	31	51%	87	57%	86	57%
Intermediate	2	1%	2	3%	2	1%	7	5%
Positive	58	44%	22	36%	52	34%	49	33%
Positive by hx	9	7%	6	10%	13	8%	7	5%
Total	133	100%	61	100%	154	100%	149	100%

Note: Heavy drinkers = ≥ 3 drinks per episode on a regular basis; light drinkers = ≤ 2 drinks occasionally, no regular drinking pattern; former drinkers = heavy drinkers in the past, light or nondrinkers now; nondrinkers = deny any alcohol use now or previously.

tained through patient interviews with data at the New York City Department of Health, Bureau of Tuberculosis. All bacteriological verifications of tuberculosis must by law be reported to the bureau. The number of old cases does not relate to the spread of the disease through the shelter population, but rather its persistance within the same people over a relatively long period of time. This group of people is important not only because of the danger to their own health posed by the persistent disease, but also because members of this group can transmit the disease to others within (and without) the shelter population.

The most striking feature of the active tuberculosis cases at Keener is the high percentage of new cases: 21 out of 26 (or 81%). Some of the individuals being treated for new active tuberculosis came to Keener with tuberculosis medications (Table 12.5, row 3), often after having been discharged from hospitals throughout New York City. However, 11 of the 26 active cases were first diagnosed while the client resided at Keener. This group (Table 12.5, row 2) to some extent shows the spread of the disease within the population of this shelter, although we cannot conclude that transmission of the disease took place within the building itself, nor even, in fact, that the disease first became active while the patient was living there. Nevertheless, the size of this group, as well as the total number of new tuberculosis cases (21 individuals), show the importance of maintaining extensive on-site medical care for the population of this shelter.

PPD Positive Individuals

There was a significantly higher PPD reactor rate among blacks (54 percent) than among whites (31 percent) or Hispanics (37 percent). (See Table 12.7.) Whether this was a function of socioeconomic status prior to arrival in the hotel/shelter system is not known. There was a significant difference in PPD reactor rates between men and women. The reason is not clear. (See Table 12.8.)

Questions were asked of each individual regarding alcohol use. We arbitrarily divided the respondents into four groups, defined in Table 12.6. Although it is difficult to determine the significance of PPD reactor rate differences between adjacent groups in this table, there appears to be a significantly higher rate in heavy drinkers, compared to non-drinkers.

Two factors in particular seemed to affect PPD reactor rates significantly: age (Table 12.9, Figure 12.2) and length of stay in shelter or SRO (Table 12.10, Figure 12.3). While the steady rise in PPD reactor rate versus age is an accepted general trend in the population of the United States at large, the prevalence in our population is three- to four-fold higher.

PPD reactor rates show a general increase with the time people spend in shelters or SROs. This suggests that living in these environments leads to dormant tuberculosis infection. To clarify this matter further, we intend to begin anniversary testing of residents with negative PPD skin tests. It is noteworthy, as Figure 12.3 indicates, that a surge of recent arrivals with positive skin tests is taking place. Many of these

Table 12.7. PPD Reactors Rate vs. Race (n = 528) (Saint Vincent's Hospital Department of Community Medicine Tuberculosis Study, September 1982– June 1984)

	White		*Black*		*Hispanic*		*Asian*		*Other*	
Negative	121	67%	125	43%	30	59%	3	75%	1	25%
Intermediate	3	2%	8	3%	2	4%	0		0	
Positive	47	26%	132	46%	12	23%	1	25%	2	50%
Positive by hx	9	5%	24	8%	7	14%	0		1	25%
Total	180	100%	289	100%	51	100%	4	100%	4	100%

Table 12.8. PPD Reactor Rate vs. Sex (n = 531)
(Saint Vincent's Hospital Department of Com-
munity Medicine Tuberculosis Study, Septem-
ber 1982–June 1984)

	Male		*Female*	
Negative	213	50%	69	65%
Intermediate	10	3%	3	3%
Positive	163	38%	32	30%
Positive by hx	39	9%	2	2%
Total	425	100%	106	100%

individuals are young men new to the Keener Shelter. They have appeared from parts unknown, already infected.

PPD reactor rates compared to education level were analyzed but we found no correlation. Although 25 percent of those questioned admitted to prior psychiatric hospitalization, there was no difference in PPD reactor rate between them and others.

Staff (n = 68) at three shelters were questioned and given skin tests. (See Table 12.11.) Staff members' overall PPD reactor rate was 38 percent. This high rate may in part be a consequence of the fact that many employees were previously shelter residents. We intend to carry out anniversary testing of staff members whose skin tests are negative.

CONCLUSIONS AND DISCUSSION

We have learned that:

1. Tuberculosis is a major problem in the SRO/homeless population of New York City.
2. Black males who spend a large amount of time in these sites are more likely to have dormant tuberculosis infection than other groups.
3. Heavy drinkers have a higher prevalence of dormant infection.
4. Staff personnel may also be at risk for developing dormant tuberculosis infection.

More demographic information needs to be gathered about the homeless population in general. If we are seeing large numbers of

Table 12.9. PPD Reactor Rate vs. Age (n = 417) (Saint Vincent's Hospital Department of Community Medicine Tuberculosis Study, September 1982–June 1984)

	Decades												
	20's		30's		40's		50's		60's		70's		80's	
Negative	68	67%	76	56%	43	55%	23	35%	16	52%	2	50%	1	100%
Intermediate	3	3%	3	2%	3	4%	2	3%	1	3%	0		0	
Positive	24	23%	52	39%	28	36%	38	57%	14	45%	2	50%	0	
Positive by hx	7	7%	4	3%	4	5%	3	5%	0		0		0	
Total	102	100%	135	100%	78	100%	66	100%	31	100%	4	100%	1	100%

Table 12.10. PPD Reactor Rate vs. Length of Stay (n=536) (Saint Vincent's Hospital Department of Community Medicine Tuberculosis Study, September 1982–June 1984)*

	1 Month or Less		2–6 Months		7–12 Months		13–24 Months		25–48 Months		49+ Months	
Negative	93	54%	61	64%	41	55%	32	47%	22	46%	33	43%
Intermediate	2	1%	1	1%	5	7%	3	4%	1	2%	0	
Positive	63	37%	28	29%	24	32%	26	38%	19	40%	37	48%
Positive by hx	14	8%	6	6%	5	7%	7	10%	6	13%	7	9%
Total	172	100%	96	100%	75	101%	68	99%	48	101%	77	100%

*Percentages that do not total 100 do so due to rounding.

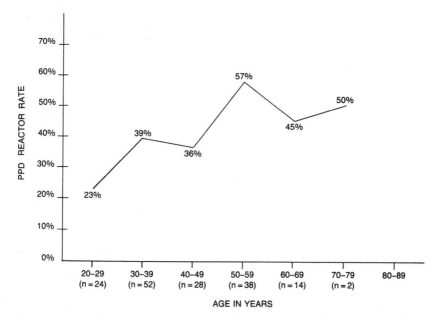

Figure 12.2. PPD Reactor Rate vs. Age (Saint Vincent's Hospital Department of Community Medicine Tuberculosis Study, September 1982–June 1984)

young people with asymptomatic tuberculosis infections who are only recently homeless and likely to return to the mainstream of society, the general health of the public may be at risk.

Now that tuberculosis is established as a major medical problem in this population, systems need to be created to ensure both that testing is done and that results are acted upon. The first phase of our study has uncovered some data that are noteworthy. The second phase will seek to define those factors that can lead to improved compliance and completion of antituberculosis therapy. Of 307 men interviewed at one site, the Keener Shelter, over an eighteen-month period, twenty-six were found to have active tuberculosis, requiring long-term therapy with two or more drugs. Of these, only eighteen remain at this site on therapy today. The numbers for follow-up of those started on INH prophylaxis during this period are worse. Of fifty persons who met the American Thoracic Society criteria for isoniazid prophylaxis, only six are still on therapy. No one has completed the requisite full year of treatment.

When this disturbing information became evident, we began to discuss the possible causes for failure. The medical charts of those indi-

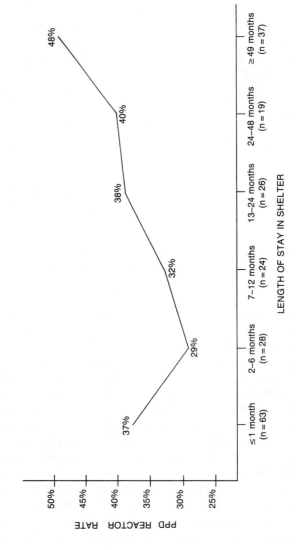

Figure 12.3. PPD Reactor Rate vs. Length of Stay (Saint Vincent's Hospital Department of Community Medicine Tuberculosis Study, September 1982–June 1984)

Table 12.11.   Staff Data; Reactor Rate by Site; Staff Only (Saint Vincent's Hospital Department of Community Medicine Tuberculosis Study, September 1982–June 1984)

	Westside Cluster		Moravian Church		Keener Building	
Negative	10	55%	6	50%	24	63%
Intermediate	2	11%	0		0	
Positive	5	28%	6	50%	13	34%
Positive by hx	1	6%	0		1	3%
Total	18	100%	12	100%	38	100%

	Total Staff	
Negative	40	59%
Intermediate	2	3%
Positive	24	35%
Positive by hx	2	3%
Total	68	100%

viduals lost to follow-up were pulled from the clinic files. All the charts told the same story: the clients had disappeared into the anonymity of the crowd. We have been able to identify cases, but we have neither the staff nor the systems to make certain that infected patients, once diagnosed, return for treatment.

We recognize that the traditional one-to-one physician–patient relationship fails in detecting and treating those at risk in this population. Medical care must be provided by teams of nursing, medical, and social work professionals. Perhaps, most importantly, the medical teams need a liaison person, such as a former shelter resident, between themselves and their clients. Thus we have begun to increase compliance for testing and follow-up by making a former client a member of the health care team. The shelter residents know and trust this person. He serves as an effective link between the staff and the residents. Also, staffing schedule changes have been made to ensure a shorter waiting time to see the doctor for tuberculosis testing and evaluation. This system seems to be working for us at one of the men's shelters.

Some of our support in obtaining compliance comes from the individuals tested. They in turn tell their comrades about the testing program. We attempt to educate as we interview. There is a wide disparity in the degree of sophistication of our patients. We have found that many do not know what tuberculosis is. As we interview and test people, we find that teaching can be done by medical team members other than the physician. A standardized checklist questionnaire, coupled with didactic sessions for team members, now produces fairly well standardized interviews. Physicians can therefore spend more of their time in patient counseling sessions for those with positive skin tests. It is through repeated contacts between the medical team members and the clients that therapeutic bonds are established.

UNRESOLVED QUESTIONS

We need to learn more; and the following major questions remain unresolved.

1. By concentrating our attention on those with active disease and giving them incentives to return for follow-up, such as choice of location of bed in the shelter, are we essentially creating new tuberculosis sanitoria? Is the problem of such magnitude that sanitoria should be reopened with inducements of safety, less crowding, cleaner surroundings, guaranteed use of medications, and better food for those who elect to have their disease treated and cured in such settings?

2. Is chronic alcohol use an absolute contraindication to isoniazid prophylaxis? Should chronic alcoholic patients be told that they should not drink if they take this medication?[10]

3. Will all these efforts result in more effective treatment of dormant and active tuberculosis? Will we truly be failing these patients if, despite our best efforts, they are unable to complete one year of traditional isoniazid prophylaxis? Even the most optimistic among us will admit that we will have failed if we cannot convince those with active tuberculosis to complete their course of therapy. But, for the greater number of patients who have only dormant infection without symptoms, will we have failed if we are not able to decrease their chance of reactivation of tuberculosis by following a regimen of isoniazid prophylaxis?

4. Will we have shown these individuals who are estranged from families, old friends, and society in general that they have worth as human beings? Can we convince them that a medical team wants to work with them, to help them to return to a state of good health, regardless of their ability to pay or ability to follow through with traditional medical regimens?

All of these are questions in urgent need of answer.

REFERENCES

1. New York City Department of Health. Tuberculosis 1882–1982. City Health Information Vol. 1, No. 22, December 8, 1982.
2. Tuberculosis–United States, 1983. MMWR, 1984; 33:412–15.
3. Slutkin G. Management of tuberculosis in urban homeless and indigent patients. Unpublished paper.
4. Sherman MN, Brickner PW, Schwartz MS, et al. Tuberculosis in single-room-occupancy hotel residents: a persisting focus of disease. NY Med Quart. Fall 1980:39–41.
5. Control of Tuberculosis. Am Rev Respir Dis. 1983; 128:2.
6. Stead WW, Bates JH. Tuberculosis. In: Petersdorf et al., eds. Harrison's Principles of Internal Medicine. 10th edition. New York: McGraw-Hill, 1983.
7. Crocco JA, Rooney JJ, Lyons HA. Outpatient treatment of tuberculosis in unreliable alcoholic patients. NY State J Med. 1976; 76:1.
8. Treatment of tuberculosis and other mycobacterial diseases. Am Rev Respir Dis. 1983; 127:6.
9. Ferebee SH. Controlled chemoprophylaxis trials in tuberculosis: a general review. Adv Tuberc Res. 1970; 17:28.
10. Kopanoff DE, Snider DE, Caras GJ. Isoniazid-related hepatitis: a U.S. Public Health Service cooperative surveillance study. Am Rev Respir Dis. 1978; 117:991.

PART III

MENTAL HEALTH AND ILLNESS

13

Psychiatry and Homelessness: Problems and Programs

Sara L. Kellermann, Ronnie S. Halper,
Marybeth Hopkins, and Gail B. Nayowith

Although there is a rapidly growing body of literature on the prevalence of psychiatric illness among homeless people, much of it is anecdotal and based on personal impressions rather than on scientific inquiry. Estimates of the number of homeless men and women who require mental health services, therefore, are no more reliable than estimates of the total number of homeless people.[1] Due to formidable obstacles in obtaining a valid sample, few systematic studies of the psychiatric status of homeless people have been conducted. Generally, the interviews or client contact sheets that comprise the data base reflect a pre-selected sample of individuals who utilize or are referred for services and exhibit behavior that staff considers indicative of mental illness.[1]

Controversy, then, continues about the incidence, prevalence, and cause of mental illness among the homeless population. Any discussion that links psychiatric illness and homeless people should also be considered within the complex interrelationships between the social, economic, and political systems that impact the lives of these individuals.

Homelessness and psychiatric illness can be viewed interactionally. Unresolved, severe psychiatric problems may result in homelessness;

conversely, homelessness may produce or exacerbate symptoms of mental illness.

CHARACTERISTICS OF THE HOMELESS

Controversial issues notwithstanding, demographic information from several recent surveys and studies provides an impression of some of the basic characteristics of this elusive population. Of some 3000 individuals screened for mental health services at shelters between February 1981 and January 1983, approximately 90 percent were male and 10 percent female. Sixty-nine percent were less than forty years of age. Ethnically, the population was found to be 31 percent black, 24 percent white, 11 percent Hispanic, and 2 percent of other ethnic origin.[2]

A 1981 survey of 107 men at the Third Street Shelter and the Keener Building, two New York City municipal shelters, revealed a median age of thirty-six years and an ethnic composition of 64 percent black, 15 percent white, and 21 percent Hispanic. Seventy percent of this group came from economically deprived backgrounds, and more than half had spent time in prison.[3]

A recent study of ninety undomiciled persons presenting at the psychiatric emergency room of Bellevue Hospital, a New York City municipal hospital, disclosed similar findings. Seventy-five percent of the sample were men. Ethnically, 38.9 percent were black; 46.7 percent, white; and 14.4 percent, Hispanic. Sixty-three percent were between twenty and thirty-nine years of age. Most impressive, however, were the findings on psychiatric hospitalization, which documented that 96.7 percent of the population had a prior history of hospitalization. Seventy-two percent had been diagnosed as schizophrenic; 13.3 percent, as having personality disorders; and 5.5 percent, as having major affective disorders. Forty-one percent acknowledged the use of drugs, alcohol, or both.[4]

Segal and Baumohl have a different schematic view of the population. They focus on the individual's social functioning and propensity to violence.[5] Their analysis describes the population as chronically dysfunctional—with minimal occupational skills and long histories of unemployment, inability to manage funds, and consistently impaired judgement in social relations. Multiple psychiatric hospitalizations are the rule, as are drug and alcohol abuse. Minor entanglements with the law are routine, often leaving the impression that criminal behavior is more pronounced than psychiatric illness. The belligerent, violent, or destructive behavior thought to result from the stresses of daily life is frequent in this population, which is further described as minimizing, projecting, or denying the responsibility or existence of psychiatric problems.[5] It is not surprising, therefore, that this group characteristically does not comply with treatment plans.

It is a commonly held belief that the depopulation of state psychiatric centers, in addition to the sociological phenomena of poverty, unemployment, and a shortage of low-cost housing, has contributed significantly to the increase in the number of mentally disabled homeless persons. Deinstitutionalization was stimulated by the advent and widespread use of psychotropic medications; legal decisions that upheld an individual's right to treatment in the least restrictive setting; attempts to maximize the federal share of state mental health expenditures through increased use of Medicaid, which does not provide reimbursement for institutionalized patients aged twenty-one to sixty-five; and professional support for the concept of community mental health and community-based care.[6,7]

The overall change in the locus of services from state psychiatric centers to neighborhood programs resulted in a census reduction in New York State facilities from 93,000 inpatients in 1955 to 20,000 in 1982. It is impossible to ascertain the number of persons discharged during that period who are currently homeless. However, the "largely unplanned" manner in which this state mental health policy was implemented indicates that a significant number of individuals returned to the community and remained there without adequate psychosocial support.[1]

A growing number of chronically mentally disabled homeless are people between the ages of eighteen and thirty-five who, prior to the implementation of admission diversion would have received long-term care in state facilities. They have been labeled "young adult chronics." The shift toward outpatient treatment, the post-World War II baby boom, and the absence of adequate community-based support services contribute to the increased visibility of these homeless young adults.

Exhibiting severe and persistent difficulties in daily functioning, young adult chronics struggle to maintain themselves in the community. Often described as volatile, impulsive, and demanding, they are very mobile and often require short stays in acute care psychiatric units. This population has been noted for its pronounced deficits in social functioning and its "tendency to use mental health services inappropriately in ways that drain the time and energy of clinicians, yet do not conform to viable treatment plans."[8] Existing, traditional mental health programs do not meet the needs of this young adult group. However, their youth and energy spark the hope that appropriate services will make a difference in their lives.

CURRENT MENTAL HEALTH PROGRAMS

Bachrach notes that programs that work for the chronic population "assign top priority to the care of the most severely impaired patients and thereby eliminate their need to compete for services; enable patients to gain access to a full range of comprehensive services; are realistically linked to other agencies and resources that assist patients; are characterized by personally designed and highly individualized services; emphasize the need for specially trained staff who are aware of the unique needs of the chronically mentally ill; show flexibility in their formats so that they may change readily in response to the changing needs of their enrollees; are tied in some manner to a complement of hospital beds; and are relevant to and compatible with the culture base in the particular communities where they are located."[8]

Three basic types of programs have been established to meet the needs of psychiatrically disabled homeless individuals: street outreach, on-site rehabilitation, and psychosocial clubs. The New York City Department of Mental Health, Mental Retardation, and Alcoholism Services administers this network of programs, which reflect the existing continuum of community care for the mentally ill homeless.

Street Outreach

Ideally, a mentally ill homeless person should be seen initially by a mobile street outreach team, engaged in treatment, referred for entitlements, and linked to a shelter. At the shelter, the individual should receive rehabilitation services from an on-site team, which would assess his or her functional potential for employment and residential options, arrange for a permanent residence in the community, and make a referral to a specialized mental health program such as a psychosocial club. The goal of services provided at a psychosocial club would be increased integration of the individual into community life.

This model of continuing progressive care, of course, does not always pertain. Individuals enter the service system in a variety of ways, and services may not always be delivered in a logically progressive and identical manner. Sufficient and appropriate resources may not exist for all clients who need them, and service coordination and linkages among provider agencies are often inadequate. In addition, the course of chronic mental illness is not linear, and it is not always appropriate to provide services to clients in a sequential fashion. Finally, it must be recognized that in a system where individuals avail themselves of services on a voluntary basis, they are free to choose the services they prefer. They can enter the system at any point and accept or reject services at any level.

Mobile street outreach programs, often the homeless individual's entry into the system, were developed to reach in an innovative and nonthreatening way chronically mentally ill persons living on the street and to help them reconnect with needed mental health and social service agencies. The initial step of the mobile outreach program involves approaching homeless individuals on the street, engaging them, and providing concrete services such as food and hygiene kits. While outreach workers try to provide supportive counseling and crisis intervention at this stage, it often takes fifteen to twenty contacts before sufficient trust has been established and basic hygiene needs met, through showers and delousing, to get to step two.[9]

In step two, the supportive counseling by the outreach workers continues. Efforts are made to secure emergency or temporary shelter and the process of applying for public assistance begins.

Securing Supplemental Security Income (SSI) benefits is the third step. Eligibility for SSI is determined by medical or psychiatric certification that the individual is unable to work because of a physical or mental disability. In an attempt to provide homeless persons with the necessary documentation, referrals may be made to a mental health agency for evaluations. For some individuals, this referral establishes an ongoing link to mental health services. For others, this linkage cannot be completed until permanent housing is obtained.

In the fourth and last step of this overall process, permanent housing is secured for these clients, and continuous encouragement to accept mental health services is provided.[9]

For some clients the relationship with the outreach program continues even after stable housing, income source, the mental health services have been secured, with the outreach workers assuming an ongoing case management role. Clients often return to the outreach program for social support or assistance when new crises arise. The process of disengagement can sometimes be as lengthy as the initial process of engagement.[9]

Crisis intervention services/psychiatric evaluations can also be provided to individuals living on the street by specialized mobile outreach teams. One such team, Project HELP, has been given permission to authorize the involuntary transport of homeless individuals who are judged to be a danger to themselves or others to a psychiatric emergency room for evaluation. It was originally anticipated that the addition of this mechanism would dramatically increase access to diagnostic and treatment services for homeless people with psychiatric emergencies.

Since its inception in October, 1982, Project HELP has made over 3800 face-to-face contacts with homeless people and has assumed responsibility for approximately 799 individuals. Over seventy people have been transported to city shelters, some forty people have been brought to hospitals or clinics for medical care, and sixteen people have been voluntarily admitted to the psychiatric inpatient unit of Bellevue Hospital. Involuntary transport authority has resulted in the admission of only seventeen cases during this period.[10]

Critical to the success of outreach services for the homeless is understanding both the timing and role of mental health referrals, which are rarely made in the early stages of the outreach process. An analysis of data of 368 psychiatrically disabled homeless clients found that outreach workers had discussed mental health services during the initial contact with only ninety-one clients, or 25 percent of the sample. Only eight of these individuals expressed a willingness to accept a psychiatric referral. An additional twelve clients were noncommittal, and seventy-one refused assistance.[9]

In several recent interviews with workers at two outreach programs, researchers were told that fear of involuntary hospitalization prevented many homeless persons from accepting any medical or psychiatric services.[9] Workers, then, must be able to tolerate the conditions under which many homeless people live and must try to avoid premature offers of mental health referrals that might jeopardize the efforts to establish a trusting relationship.[9] Further exploration of the general efficacy of street outreach teams to provide involuntary treatment to homeless people will continue.

On-Site Rehabilitation

Another type of program, on-site rehabilitation services in the form of psychosocial skill development groups, was specifically designed to serve individuals who were functionally disabled due to mental illness; that is, individuals unable to perform age- and role-appropriate tasks of daily living and either unwilling or unable to utilize traditional mental health services. Increased independent functioning was expected to result if services were provided at the person's residence. On-site rehabilitation programs were, therefore, established at a number of congregate care facilities such as shelters, private proprietary homes for adults, and single-room-occupancy (SRO) residences.

In addition to mental health clinic services, this model includes socialization groups, which focus on such topics as travel training, budgeting, nutrition, prevocational skills training, grooming, and self-care. These socialization activities are offered as a means of reacquainting homeless individuals with activities that are an integral part of community life. Such groups may also focus on work and leisure, education, and interpersonal relationships.

Nearly all of the people served by on-site rehabilitation programs have histories of psychiatric hospitalization. Frequently, after-care plans made prior to discharge were either inappropriate, inadequate, or nonexistent, and the individuals wound up in the shelter system. The security of a bed and three meals a day at the shelter often enables clients, with the help of staff, to work toward stabilized psychiatric conditions and improved social functioning.

Rehabilitation programs assist individuals in controlling psychopathological symptoms and in developing more effective coping mechanisms. The goals of treatment include improved social relations and overall individual functioning. A good rehabilitation program clarifies clients' expectations about the degrees of dependence and independence that they can tolerate.[11]

Some individuals may be unable to tolerate placement in a permanent residence. For them, the goals of rehabilitation programs are modified somewhat to take individual limitations into account. The possibility of eventual community placement, however, is never foreclosed. Often these individuals experience an institutional transference to the shelter setting, and the idea of moving creates tremendous anxiety. In these instances, the goal is to maintain the individuals in the program and promote the development of skills that will afford the highest possible quality of life.

Individuals capable of moving from an on-site rehabilitation program in a shelter to a permanent residence in the community may be referred to a community-based mental health service provider. Clients able to connect to a new agency are assisted during this transitional period through intensive case management and follow-up services by the former service agency, to ensure a successful referral.

Psychosocial Clubs

Another treatment model, the psychosocial club, provides services that are similar to those of an on-site rehabilitation program. Clients who attend such programs in the community ostensibly function on a higher level than those using on-site rehabilitation services in shelters. Such group treatment tends to be effective and can help to establish a therapeutic community. Here, the primary goal is to encourage individuals to move from social isolation to social interaction.[12]

RECOMMENDATIONS

These program models have met with reasonable success in addressing the needs of mentally ill homeless people. It should be noted, however, that a proportion of psychiatrically disabled homeless people will reject available services of any kind. The service system presently offers few mental health services to these people that will make a difference in the quality of their lives, particularly in the absence of appropriate housing resources. It is unclear whether individual pathology or the unavailability of appropriate services is at the root of the problem, but the question of how these individuals differ from homeless people who use services must be addressed through continued research.

While community-based day programs such as psychosocial clubs work well with the psychiatrically disabled homeless, it must be emphasized that a client's ability to achieve his or her highest functional level is compromised in the absence of residential options. An intermediate level of care is needed to prepare these individuals both to accept ongoing mental health treatment services and to function independently at their maximum capacity.[1] A long-term transitional housing program is required for the homeless who are chronically mentally disabled. The aim of such a program would be to secure permanent housing and treatment for each resident. In order to maintain a residential atmosphere and not that of a psychiatric center, each resident would receive mental health and supportive social services from an off-site community-based provider. The program would be staffed by psychiatrists, registered nurses, social workers, rehabilitation counselors, occupational and activities therapists, home economists, rehabilitation aides, and case managers.[1] Grooming and self-care skills would be emphasized by residence staff, as would social skills and such practical skills as shopping, housekeeping, cooking, traveling, and managing money. Transportation would be provided in order to maximize access to recreational and other community resources. Vocational rehabilitation and job placement services would also be made available.

In a recent cooperative effort between the New York City Human

Resources Administration and the State Office of Mental Health, a shelter for psychiatrically disabled homeless individuals, the Queens Shelter Care Center for Men, has been established on the campus of Creedmoor Psychiatric Center. Plans are under development to establish a domiciliary care facility for this population on the same campus. The domiciliary care facility represents an interim step toward the development of the transitional housing model previously mentioned. A clinic treatment program and a continuing treatment program are currently being developed with a voluntary mental health provider to serve clients in these facilities. These resources represent an important first step toward the establishment of discrete shelter units for the psychiatrically disabled homeless. It is hoped that future programs will expand upon this initiative, establishing smaller-scale residences with programs designed and staffed to offer the intensive rehabilitation services needed by the chronically mentally disabled homeless population.

Finally, the development of low-cost housing options in the community is essential to long-range efforts to provide mental health services to homeless people. The operation and administration of SRO hotels, such as the Saint Francis Residence in Manhattan, or of scatter-site apartment programs would be consistent with efforts to rehabilitate and treat mentally ill homeless persons in the community.

CONCLUSION

The mentally ill homeless population is heterogeneous, as are their mental health needs. Continued identification of those variables that lead to the mitigation of the condition of homelessness is crucial to efforts to plan and establish appropriate services. Program effectiveness must be evaluated, with emphasis given to the kinds of models that work for specific subgroups of the chronically mentally ill homeless.

Access to long-and short-term psychiatric hospitalization should be ensured for needy individuals, as should the creation of a range of appropriate treatment programs. Professional, educational, or monetary incentives to treat chronically mentally ill disabled homeless persons should be initiated for clinical treatment staff.

Finally, the dialogues that have begun between housing, social service, mental health, and health agencies must be formalized and continued if the problem of homelessness is to be successfully addressed and ultimately prevented.

REFERENCES

1. Mental health plan for homeless adults in New York City. New York City Department of Mental Health, Mental Retardation and Alcoholism Services, Bureau of Rehabilitation and Special Services and Office of Planning and Project Management. Supplement to the NYC Human Resources Administration Comprehensive Plan for Community Support Services Funds Submitted September 11, 1981: November 30, 1981.
2. New York State Office of Mental Health shelter outreach project statistical report—two years at the shelters. New York State Office of Mental Health, New York Regional Office, February 1981 to January 1983.
3. Hoffman SP, Wenger D, Nigro J, Rosenfeld R. Who are the homeless? a study of randomly selected men who use the New York City shelters. New York State Office of Mental Health, New York Regional Office, 1982.
4. Lipton FR, Sabatini A, Katz SE. Down and out in the city: the homeless mentally ill. Hospital and Community Psychiatry. 1983; 34(9):817–21.
5. Segal SP, Baumohl J. Engaging the disengaged: proposals on madness and vagrancy. Social Work. 1980; September: 359.
6. Jurow GL. Financing long term care for the chronically mentally impaired in New York State: an issue analysis. Issued by State Communities Aid Association Institute on Care of the Mentally Impaired in the Long Term Care System 1979.
7. From country asylums to city streets: the contradiction between deinstitutionalization and state mental health funding priorities. Office of New York City's Council President Carol Bellamy. Prepared by Cindy Lynn Freidmutter, Esq., June 1979.
8. Bachrach, LL. Program planning for young adult chronic patients. In: Pepper B, Ryglewicz H, eds.The young adult chronic patient. Vol. 14. San Francisco: Jossey-Bass, 1982:99–109.
9. Barrow S, Lovell A. The referral of outreach clients to mental health services. The Community Support Systems Evaluation Program at New York State Psychiatric Institute.
10. Project H.E.L.P. Summary Statistics—A CSS-Funded Project at Gouvernuer Hospital: March 12–18. New York City Health and Hospital Corporation, 1984.
11. Christmas JJ. Group rehabilitative approaches in socially and economically disadvantaged communities. In: Sager CJ, Kaplan HS, eds. Progress in group and family therapy. New York: Brunner/Mazel, 1972.
12. Christmas JJ, Daniels MS. A socio-psychiatric approach to rehabilitation in a low-income community. Presented at the fifth annual national meeting of the Psychiatric Outpatient Centers of America, Washington, DC, 1967.

14

The Toll
of Deinstitutionalization

Kevin Flynn

The homeless are the unemployed, the bag ladies, the runaways, the abandoned children known as "pushouts," the alcoholics, the drug abusers, the new immigrants. The mentally ill make up a substantial proportion of the homeless. The streets of our cities have become the abode of hundreds of thousands of mentally disturbed individuals who are either former state mental hospital patients, applicants to state hospitals who have been rejected due to rigid restrictions, or simply those on whom street life has taken its toll. In every part of the United States, we have witnessed a major increase in the number of homeless in recent years. In Philadelphia alone, for instance, the number of individuals living in emergency family housing increased fivefold between 1981 and 1983. Agencies such as the Salvation Army have noted significant increases in the number of persons seeking emergency assistance. Madeline R. Stoner notes that more women, elderly and young people, particularly black women and other minorities, have joined the older, alcoholic white men on our skid rows.[1]

DEINSTITUTIONALIZATION

As Fustero noted recently in *Psychology Today*:

> Approximately one-third to one-half of the homeless are believed
> to be mentally ill and on the streets primarily because of a process
> known as deinstitutionalization which was initiated more than
> twenty years ago when thousands of patients began to be released
> from state mental hospitals.[2]

In 1960, 535,000 psychiatric patients were living in state hospitals
in the United States. By 1980 the number had dropped to 137,000. In
California, deinstitutionalization reduced the state psychiatric population from 37,000 in 1955 to only 2500 in 1983.[3]

At the same time, state mental institutions initiated extremely restrictive admission policies, making reentry virtually impossible. The
mentally disturbed now move precariously from hospitals to slums to
jails in a "revolving door syndrome." Approximately 18 percent of the
patients in the Forensic Inpatient Program in Los Angeles County Jail
were either from or heading toward skid row.[4]

Deinstitutionalization presumed that funds would be available to
create programs that would provide for the mental health needs of
former and future patients. For the thousands of discharged psychiatric
patients who ended up in the slums of our cities, the promised funds
never arrived and the urgently needed range of psychiatric services in
the community failed to evolve. The discharged patients were, in effect, abandoned and found themselves outside the mainstream of
American life.

Uri Aviram and Steven Segal point to the exclusion of the mentally
ill in society.

> Physical exclusion by removal of the mentally ill from certain resi-
> dential areas or by blocking their entrance is an indication of com-
> munity resistance to the integration of the mentally ill. Communities
> have used various tactics both formal and informal in the mani-
> festation of this resistance. We have also noted that in many cases
> where the mentally ill are in the community they are socially ex-
> cluded either by mechanisms that foster a docility or by forces that
> encourage ghettoization. It should indeed be determined if the dy-
> namic of exclusion which kept the mentally ill in the back wards
> of the hospitals will relegate them to the back alleys of the
> community.[5]

In their study, Reich and Siegel found "on the Bowery and at the Men's Shelter . . . a microcosm of the former State Hospital system. The intervention unit resembles feature-for-feature the old prototype situation—with patients wandering, hallucinating, and aimlessly shifting about."[6]

The Departments of Health and Human Services and Housing and Urban Development summarize the problem very well in a report:

> Finally, there are increasing numbers of chronically mentally ill individuals among the homeless. These are most visible in urban settings and may be seen in public places—on sidewalks, on park benches, in subways, train stations, and bus depots. A small minority of them are able to secure a bed for the night in such emergency housing alternatives as public or private shelters or church missions. Others may occasionally spend the night in flophouses or Bowery-type hotels. For the most part, however, they sleep for short intervals in public areas.
>
> . . . Therefore, the information suggests that nationwide several tens of thousands of chronically mentally ill individuals have no housing whatsoever. Current data on emergency shelters of all types indicate that such programs are meeting the needs of less than 10 percent of the homeless population.[7]

THE RELATIONSHIP OF HOMELESSNESS, MENTAL HEALTH, AND POVERTY

Fried acknowledges a relationship between poverty and mental disorders:

> The evidence is unambiguous and powerful that the lowest social classes have the highest rate of psychiatric disorder in our society. Regardless of the measures employed for estimating severe psychiatric disorder and social class, regardless of the region or the date of study and regardless of the method of study the great majority of results all point clearly and strongly to the fact that the lowest social class has by far the greatest incidence of psychosis.
>
> . . . At the very least most of the forms of situational stress, for example marital disruption, migration and forced residential relocation, physical illness and unemployment, occur with disproportionate frequency among lower class populations. . . . If these bear any relationship to the occurrence of mental disorder, we can expect higher rates of psychiatric disorder regardless of the extrin-

sic influences that make them more visible or that translate malfunctioning into psychiatric disorder and hospitalization.[8]

Miller and Mishler conducted a study of mental health and social
class structure in New Haven, Connecticut, and concluded that the
lower classes comprise two-thirds of that community and contribute
more than three-fourths of its mental patients. The proportion of patients diagnosed as psychotic is disproportionately represented in the
lower class.[9] In addition, people with emotional problems tend to drift
down in social class, a view held by Fried:

> Despite reservations we can tentatively conclude that the hypoth-
> esis that individuals with severe psychiatric disorders show either
> disproportionate low rates of upward mobility or disproportionate
> high rates of downward mobility is sustained.
>   There is also evidence to indicate that in some instances, prob-
> ably something less than a majority, experiences of unemployment
> are significant causal factors leading to disorganization and psy-
> chiatric disorder.[8]

Cohn conducted a longitudinal study between 1968 and 1973 in
which he sampled 5000 heads of families. Those who became unemployed and reemployed were compared with individuals who remained
employed. He concluded that job loss was associated with negative self-
concept, which for many persisted after reemployment.[10] Braginsky
similarly found a dramatic loss of self-esteem among those who had
experienced job loss.[11] Brenner found a statistically significant relationship between unemployment and suicide, state prison admissions,
homicide, and mortality.[12]

Among the poor, unemployment often results in a loss of residence, the individual's support network, and sense of community. This
alienation experienced by the homeless is a chronic condition that often
removes them from the goods, services, and supports of our society.

Miller has developed a model that relates family stability with economic stability. He defines four categories:[13]

1. Stable Poor: Characterized by stability both economically and
within the family. Regularly employed, low-skilled.

2. Strained: Typified by a secure economic pattern but an unstable
family that may include wild younger members or older alcoholic
parents who disturb family functioning.

3. Coping: Defined by economic insecurity and family stability.
This group probably increases during periods of extensive layoffs.

4. Unstable: Characterized by neither economic nor family stability. There are degrees of instability within this group.

Miller states that, "The low-income class generally and the unstable in particular is a category of unskilled, irregular workers, broken and large families, and a residual bin of the aged, physically handicapped, and mentally disturbed."[13]

In relating the plight of the homeless to this matrix, it is evident that the strained, the coping, and the unstable subgroups are heavily represented in the homeless population. Those who experience economic insecurity, the coping and the unstable, are the first to feel the negative effects of a depressed economy and end up on the streets. People in the strained category may find that their unstable family constellation disintegrates as a result of the traditional stress of layoffs or the threat of job loss. When the family breaks up, a significant number of women and children become homeless. We can see the powerful effects of economic factors on economically insecure groups as well as on emotionally unstable families. Those who have neither economic nor family stability are the most likely to become homeless and the most emotionally vulnerable to the wretched experience of attempting to survive on the streets.

MENTAL HEALTH OF THE HOMELESS

Dr. William Mayer testified before a U.S. Senate Subcommittee:

> It is not possible to provide accurate national data on homelessness. But we do know that the homeless population in this country is not a homogeneous one; that it includes runaway children, immigrants, migrants, so-called bag ladies, the recently evicted, certain numbers of the unemployed, battered women, and an overrepresentation of minorities. We also know that the problems and characteristics of this population vary according to locality.[14]

Dr. Mayer conservatively estimates that between 35 and 40 percent of homeless persons have a primary alcohol, drug abuse, or mental disorder.[14]

A number of recent studies have focused on psychiatric needs and profiles of street people.

In Los Angeles County, Skid Row Project was the way-station for discharged mental patients from state hospitals, private hospitals, and prisons. An estimated 40 percent of the males and 90 percent of the females in Skid Row Project had serious mental disorders. In addition, 40 percent of the males and 15 to 20 percent of the females had serious alcohol or other drug dependencies.[15] Ed Eisenstadt, director of the Volunteers of America Weingart Multiservice Center in Los Angeles, estimates that up to 50 percent of the homeless in skid row suffer from alcohol or other drug problems.

Arce and colleagues[16] report that 35 percent of all shelter residents indicated previous psychiatric treatment in state hospitals, psychiatric units in the community, or Veterans Administration hospitals. Previous treatment in alcohol or drug detoxification programs was reported by 4.7 percent. When residents were evaluated using the criteria set forth in the *Diagnostic and Statistical Manual of Mental Disorders,*[17] 84 percent of the residents were diagnosed as having some mental illness. Schizo-phrenia was the primary diagnosis in 34 percent, substance abuse in 25 percent, personality disorder in 7 percent, affective disorder in 6 per-cent, and organic brain syndrome or other disorder in 5 percent. A secondary diagnosis of substance abuse appeared in 18 percent of the residents, and mental retardation in 1 percent. Thus 43 percent had ma-jor problems with alcohol or other drug abuse. This proportion sup-ports the conclusions of Blumberg, Shipley, and Shandler, who studied men on Philadelphia's skid row in 1966 and found 35 percent to be pathological or uncontrolled drinkers.[18]

Shelter surveys conducted by Baxter and Hopper[19] showed that psychiatric problems rivaled alcoholism as the predominant disorder of homeless men. Fifty to 70 percent of the homeless men showed some psychiatric problem, and 31 percent to 74 percent had histories of psy-chiatric hospitalization. The majority of homeless women were under forty years of age, and 58.5 percent had histories of psychiatric hos-pitalization; 13 percent had come to the shelters directly from hospitals.

Lipton, Sabatini, and Katz report that approximately 50 percent of the homeless in New York suffer significant mental disability. At New York's Bellevue Hospital the number of homeless patients who have been admitted for care has more than doubled over the past three years.[20]

Reich and Siegel report that organic mental syndrome is the most frequent psychiatric disorder in Bowery men over the age of forty. However, those under forty (more than 55 percent of the Bowery popu-lation) most frequently present paranoid schizophrenia and severe per-sonality disturbance, either alone or in combination. Many Vietnam veterans were noted on the Bowery.[6] These young adults are typically male and highly transient. Traditional mental health programs have reported significant difficulties in working with this population.[21]

While homeless people are also at risk with regard to physical illness, Fried points out:

> . . . recent histories of severe or protracted illness more frequent among the lowest status groups color the experience of mental illness and may more often initiate psychological disorganization among lower-class people.[8]

The Experience of Homelessness

The experience of being homeless gives the best context within which to understand the psychology of the homeless. John R. Coleman, President of the Edna McConnell Clark Foundation, is recognized for his work investigating the lives of the disadvantaged. After spending ten days on the streets of New York in the middle of winter, he described the Men's Shelter at 8 East 3rd Street:

> I've seen plenty of drawings of London's workhouses and asylums in the times of Charles Dickens. Now I've seen the real thing, in the last years of the twentieth century in the world's greatest city.
> The lobby and the adjacent "sitting room" were jammed with men standing, sitting, or stretched out in various positions on the floor. It was as lost a collection of souls as I could have imagined. Old and young, scarred and smooth, stinking and clean, crippled and hale, drunk and sober, ranting and still, parts of another world and parts of this one. The city promises to take in anyone who asks. Those rejected everywhere else find their way to East 3rd Street.[22]

The Feeling of Powerlessness

Powerlessness goes hand in hand with hopelessness. Those who feel powerless generally have a sense of inadequacy, loss, and inability to control their own destiny. Reduced self-esteem is tied to a lack of control over one's fate. It is reasonable to expect a high degree of psychiatric disorder among people who must depend upon forces external to themselves.[8]

The sense of powerlessness experienced by homeless people is severe. They are relegated to the back streets of our society, where they are preyed upon by unscrupulous landlords, robbers known as jackrollers, and murderers. Many homeless women report incidents of desertion as well as emotional, physical, and sexual abuse. Runaway children and pushouts are the most vulnerable to victimization on the streets. Many are the prey of "chickenhawks," pimps who beat, rob, rape, sodomize, and force them into prostitution and drug abuse.

The homeless are constantly reminded of their lack of control over virtually any aspect of their lives. Overworked bureaucrats are often insensitive to their plight. A forty-year-old woman, who had always functioned in marginal jobs, was laid-off during the recent economic recession and subsequently lost her small apartment. She stored her possessions with a commercial storage company and moved to a downtown mission. She applied for welfare and sought employment. When the storage rental bill came due, the company informed her that they would auction her goods at 1:00 P.M. that day. She appealed to the Welfare Department for her check and was told that it would not be issued until late that afternoon. She frantically returned to the rental storage company and asked for a three-hour extension. The company refused, auctioned her goods, then issued her a check, for approximately $24, for the amount above her bill. Later that afternoon the Welfare Department issued a check to the lady.

This woman did not choose her condition. Homelessness is not a matter of choice. Reports from every sector support the conclusion that when homeless people are offered safe, appropriate shelter they are eager to accept, as Baxter and Hopper found:

> Where decent, humane shelter has been made available, it has never lacked willing recipients. In light of this finding, one may be moved to wonder whether the presumption of incompetence on the part of the disabled indigent has not more the character of self-fulfilling prophecy than it does that of a faithful reporting of the "facts."[19]

Yoosuf Haveliwala, former chief executive officer of the Creedmoor Psychiatric Center, goes further:

> When these people [the mentally ill] find themselves in a city shelter, the entire mental health system has failed because many of the shelters are little more than the back wards of the past, when only custodial services were offered in our mental hospitals. What is happening, yet we fail to admit it, is that we are reverting back to warehousing psychiatric patients. If one has seen the Creedmoor shelter, "warehouse" is the appropriate word.[23]

TREATMENT PROGRAMS

Treatment programs for the mentally ill homeless need to address every facet of their life experience.

Basic Needs

Mental health needs can only be provided in a setting that ensures that the patients' basic physical needs are also addressed. The most critical need is shelter. Programs that separate mental health issues from basic needs are doomed to failure.

Employment

The Skid Row Development Corporation in Los Angeles offers financial incentives to businesses to encourage them to move into the area and to hire inner city residents. The Salvation Army also addresses the need for employment through its rehabilitation programs. In a unique cooperative effort with the Midnight Mission in Los Angeles, the California Department of Human Resources has set up one of their employment offices at the mission.

Reaching Out to the Mentally Ill

Mental health programs must seek out those in need. Proper staffing and resources are crucial. Mental health teams should operate in conjunction with other health professionals and consult with missions, single-room-occupancy hotels (SROs) and service providers. Programs must be accessible to the target clients and should be established within walking distance of the areas where the homeless are concentrated. The Los Angeles Skid Row project office was located in a skid row welfare building. The director and staff spent time with clients on the street, in the soup kitchens, schools, community centers, and in the missions.

The Weingart Center, in the heart of skid row in Los Angeles, is a multiservice center. A mental health unit and a health department clinic are but two of the programs located there, making simple the coordination between the alcoholism services provided by the Volunteers of America and the Public Inebriate Program. In recognition of the large numbers of veterans among the homeless, the Veterans Administration has offices in the center as well as a comprehensive treatment program in the skid row area. Finally, short-term housing is also available in the center.

Angel's Flight in Los Angeles is an excellent example of a program that outreaches to its clients to prevent mental health problems. Runners seek out runaway youths at the downtown bus depot and on the streets before pimps can reach these homeless children. Angel's Flight and other programs that address the problems of the homeless youth, such as Children of the Night in Hollywood and Covenant House in New York, provide shelter and counseling and do daily battle with pimps seeking "their property."

Therapeutic Relationships

The manner of approach in working with this population should communicate equality, respect, and dignity. The homeless may have had negative experiences with the mental health system in the past and will be appropriately distrustful of our intentions. Mental health professionals may validly make their first contact as simple as introducing themselves and handing the potential client a business card, while explaining their availability in the community.

Professionals need to develop trust and to build relationships with the mentally ill homeless. Patience is crucial. Every effort should be made to ensure the patient's sense of autonomy, quality, and control in any interaction.

The homeless need to feel safe. They are pragmatic and action oriented. Abstractions are not relevant to them. They are externally oriented because their world is precarious. Their deliberative processes are slow and cautious.

The Downtown Women's Center, founded and directed by Jill Halverson, is a refuge for chronically homeless women in the Los Angeles inner city. This program reaches out to vulnerable women and, through a caring, family-styled program, establishes a relationship based upon trust and dignity. No questions are asked and no forms are required. The women feel a sense of belonging and are active participants in every phase of the program that includes food, shelter, clothing, bathing facilities, health, and mental health services.

Coordination of Community Resources

The coordination of community resources is also essential. Timely clinical intervention through the cooperation of all providers of care to the homeless is possible and is beneficial to patient and provider alike. In 1981 Concerned Agencies Metropolitan Los Angeles (CAMLA) was formed to help coordinate services to the Los Angeles homeless. CAMLA published a service directory and issues copies to agencies in and outside of skid row. CAMLA helps maximize the available services and acts as an advocate for the residents of the "hospital without walls." Professionals need to be aware of all available services in order effectively to connect clients with the services they most need.

Many of the mentally ill homeless are entitled to financial assistance, such as welfare, Supplemental Security Income, and Veterans Administration entitlements, yet they are unable to negotiate the complex bureaucratic maze without assistance. In addition, identification requirements are unrealistic for this population, whose possessions are often stolen, damaged, or lost. The establishment of mental health service offices at the missions, welfare agencies, and clinics offers the mentally ill person opportunity to connect with the greater social service support network. In Los Angeles many mentally ill persons are eligible for reduced fare bus passes; a mental health professional need only fill out the form, which takes but a few minutes.

In addition, clients who are unable to follow all the social service rules and regulations should not be cut from welfare. Considering the mental health problems in this population, it should be presumed that the individual cannot comply and should therefore not be terminated from services until a mental health evaluation has been performed.

Homeless people can be empowered through coalitions and advocates. In December 1983 a coalition of lawyers that included the Legal Aid Foundation and Inner City Law Center filed a lawsuit to force the County of Los Angeles Department of Public Social Service to issue temporary housing vouchers to all eligible applicants, including those with no identification. In my capacity as a psychologist, I was asked to write a deposition dealing with the mentally traumatic effects of homelessness. Through such depositions the attorneys were able to bring to the attention of the courts the plight of the homeless in concrete terms. The court issued a restraining order and homeless people in Los Angeles County, including those with no identification, are currently issued daily housing vouchers or checks for eight dollars. This is an example of how mental health professionals can work in conjunction with other professionals to benefit the homeless mentally ill.

Traditional Patterns of Psychiatric Treatment for the Poor

Individuals from the lower class, which includes the mentally ill homeless, when compared with other classes, have not fared well at the hands of the mental health system in the United States. According to

Miller and Mishler,[9] the source of treatment referrals varies systematically by social class. Among upper-class (Class I) psychotics, one-third
of the patients were self-referred and another 40 percent came to treatment through family and friends. For working-class psychotics (Class
IV), police and court referrals accounted for 19 percent of the cases,
while in the lower class (Class V), these two sources accounted for 52
percent of the patients in treatment and social agencies accounted for
20 percent. The findings for schizophrenia are similar to those found
for psychosis in general. Miller and Mishler note that:

> There is a definite tendency to induce disturbed persons in Class
> I and Class II (the upper classes) to see a psychiatrist in more gen-
> tle and "insightful" ways than is the practice in Class IV (the work-
> ing class) and especially in Class V (the lower class), where direct
> authoritative, compulsory and at times coercively brutal methods
> are used.[9]

Schaffer and Myers[24] hypothesized that mentally ill patients, regardless of their social class, would receive intensive individual psychotherapy if economic factors were eliminated. In a 1954 study, they
found that social class did seem to play a role. Not only were patients
from upper social classes accepted for individual treatment more often,
but the patient was more apt to be seen by a more senior or more experienced member of the staff than was the case for patients from lower
social classes. A UCLA Medical Center study confirmed that social class
was a factor in the level of acceptance for psychotherapy even when
cost was eliminated as a variable.[25]

Fanshel reported that "social workers' evaluations of the treatability
of clients is inversely related to the social class position of clients."[26]
Hollingshead and Redlich also "found real differences in where, how,
and how long persons in the several classes have been cared for by psychiatrists."[27] Miller and Mishler conclude that

> the needs of the population for psychiatric treatment were not be-
> ing met adequately. What this investigation demonstrates beyond
> this is that the distribution of available resources is socially dis-
> criminatory. We believe that a serious moral question is also in-
> volved in this discovery, since the psychiatric profession legitimates
> its claim to high status and to economic and social rewards on the
> grounds that it functions in a "universalistic" nondiscriminatory
> way. Actually it operates in such a way as to restrict its "best" treat-
> ment to persons of the upper social class.[9]

Support Services to Other Service Providers

There is a need for mental health professionals to act in consultation with all providers of services to the homeless. This helps the providers understand and better serve the homeless and anticipate and avoid personnel burnout. Mental health professionals should also be represented on the boards of directors of nonprofit and community agencies that serve the homeless to advise on the needs of the mentally ill homeless.

Burnout

It is difficult to find mental health professionals to work among the homeless. Therefore every effort should be made to reduce the incidence of burnout among those who volunteer their energies to this work. Symptoms of burnout can include an elevated level of cynicism toward the bureaucracy and a hardened attitude towards the suffering of the individuals being served.

Ford Kuramoto, Director of Hollywood Mental Services, initiated a program to reduce burnout among the staff at Hollywood Mental Health Center. The program, known as the Quality of Work Life Groups, emphasizes timely cooperative problem solving among all levels of staff. It particularly encourages constructive staff interaction; different groups work on different problems and report back to the whole staff. The process greatly improves morale by enabling everyone to have a more meaningful effect on the organization.

Orientation programs should focus on dispelling irrational fears held by many who have not worked in the slums of our cities. Many fear predators, mentally disturbed people, lice, rats, disease, and a host of other hazards. Through group discussion, presentations by those who work in the area, and education regarding normal precautions, many of the irrational fears can be alleviated. Many fear for their safety in going to and coming from the work site. However, those who prey on the vulnerable homeless avoid confrontation with service providers because they know it is safer to pick on a powerless person than one who has the backing of a powerful agency. Another area of concern is the management of disruptive behavior. Staff can be trained to work in close harmony as a team to deal effectively with potentially violent individuals.

SUMMARY

The problems of the homeless mentally ill are varied and complex. We have seen how innovative programs situated in the heart of the areas where the homeless congregate are successful in reaching out to the mentally ill. In addition, the coordination of services to the homeless can maximize limited resources. Decent shelter is the most basic need. Treatment programs must be flexible and tailored to the unique needs of this population. Finally, we all need to be aware of the high risk of burnout in working with the most disadvantaged in our society, and steps should be taken to maintain and enhance our own mental health.

REFERENCES

1. Stoner MR. An analysis of public and private sector provisions for homeless people. Soc Policy. March 1984.
2. Fustero S. Home on the street. Psychology Today. February 1984:57–63.
3. DeRisi W, Vega WA. The impact of deinstitutionalization on California's state hospital population. Hosp & Comm Psych. 1983; 34:140.
4. Chen PL. Personal communication (director, Inpatient Program). Los Angeles, 1983.
5. Aviram U, Segal S. Exclusion of the mentally ill: reflection on an old problem in a new context. Arch Gen Psych. 1973; 29:131.
6. Reich R, Siegel L. The emergence of the Bowery as a psychiatric dumping ground. Psychiatric Quarterly. 1978; 50:3.
7. U.S., Department of Health and Human Services and Department of Housing and Urban Development. Report on federal efforts to respond to the shelter and basic living needs of chronically mentally ill individuals. February 1983.
8. Fried M. Social differences in mental health. In: Kosa J, Antonovsky A, Zola IK, eds. Poverty and health: a sociological analysis. Cambridge, Mass.: Harvard University Press, 1969.
9. Miller SM, Mishler EG. Social class, mental illness and American psychiatry: an expository review. In: Riessman F, Cohen J, Pearl A, eds. Mental health of the poor. Glencoe: The Free Press of Glencoe, Collier-MacMillan Ltd, 1964:16–36.
10. Cohn RM. The effect of employment change on self attitudes. Soc Psychology. 1978; 41:81–93.
11. Braginsky DD, Braginsky BM. Surplus people: their lost faith in self and system. Psychology Today. August 1975:69–72.
12. Brenner MH. Estimating the social costs of national economic policy. Study prepared for the Joint Economic Committee, US Congress, 1976.
13. Miller SM. The American lower class: a typological approach. In: Riess-

man F, Cohen J, Pearl A, eds. Mental health of the poor. Glencoe: The Free Press of Glencoe, Collier-MacMillan Ltd., 1964.

14. U.S., Congress, Senate, Subcommittee on District of Columbia Appropriations. Testimony of Mayer W. 98th Congress, 24 January 1983.
15. Farr R. The Los Angeles skid row mental health project. Los Angeles County Department of Mental Health, 1982.
16. Arce AA, Tadlock M, Vergare M, Shapiro S. A psychiatric profile of street people admitted to an emergency shelter. Hosp & Comm Psych. 1983; 34:812.
17. American Psychiatric Association: Diagnostic and Statistical Manual of Mental Disorders. 3rd edition. 1980.
18. Blumberg L, Shipley TE, Shandler IW. The development, major goals and strategies of a skid row program. Quart J Stud Alcohol. 1966; 27:242-58.
19. Baxter E, Hopper K. Private lives, public spaces: homeless adults on the streets of New York City. New York: Community Service Society of New York, 1981.
20. Lipton F, Sabatini A, Katz S. Down and out in the city: the homeless mentally ill. Hosp & Comm Psych. 1983; 34:817-21.
21. Schwartz S, Goldfinger S. The new chronic patient: clinical characteristics of an emerging subgroup. Hosp & Comm Psych. 1981; 32:470-74.
22. Coleman JR. Diary of a homeless man. New York Magazine. February 21, 1983:32.
23. Haveliwala Y. Treating the mentally ill homeless. New York Times, February 29, 1984:A22.
24. Schaffer L, Myers J. Psychotherapy and social stratification. Psychiatry. 1954; 17:83-89.
25. Brill N, Storrow H. Social class and psychiatric treatment. In: Riessman F, Cohen J, Pearl A, eds. Mental health of the poor. Glencoe: The Free Press of Glencoe, Collier-MacMillan Ltd, 1964.
26. Fanshel D: A study of caseworkers. Social Casework. 1958; 39:543-51.
27. Hollingshead A, Redlich F. Social class and mental illness. New York: John Wiley & Sons, 1958.

15

Psychiatric Care for the Homeless: Human Beings or Cases?

Litrelle T. Levy and Barbara Henley

Convention holds that approximately 40 percent of the homeless are in need of ongoing psychiatric care.[1] Individuals who are homeless, who lose their locus of security and identity, are likely to manifest psychiatric disorders sooner or later. It should be our goal to humanize the scope and quality of the mental health services available to these people.

THE TEMPORARILY HOMELESS

Housing for people who become temporarily homeless as a result of natural disaster or sweeping catastrophe is almost unquestionably forthcoming. The temporarily homeless will be accommodated as well as their families, churches, neighbors, insurance policies, or public agencies can afford. For the short haul all support systems are primed, programmed, and sustained by reasonable expectations that matters will work out. Crises of temporary deprivation validate and reinforce one's belief system and characteristic coping skills. Thus the very essence of one's societal base is paradoxically both threatened and perpetuated by the temporary homelessness that results from calamity.

Disaster victims often experience psychiatric symptoms that render them mildly to totally dysfunctional. Public education has decreased resistance to acknowledging psychiatric symptoms such as nightmares, insomnia, inability to concentrate, or survivor guilt. This change in attitudes enables mental health professionals to prescribe and deliver treatment more successfully.

In 1983, a Gulf Coast community was devastated by hurricane Alicia.[2] Local mental health agencies were granted federal funds to: (1) educate victims, their friends, neighbors, teachers, ministers, hair dressers, general medical practitioners, and others to recognize signs of posttraumatic stress syndrome, and (2) provide psychotherapeutic intervention, such as direct treatment, supervision, and consultation, based on the assumption that existing treatment capacity would have been already overloaded. The successful brief treatment for behaviors perceived as unusual—from merely bothersome to abnormal and frightening—begins with the recognition that they are an expected, typical sequel to great stress, thus converting the isolating, symptom-escalating fear from "I must be going crazy" to "at least I'm not alone." Overall, this use of public funds to expose and meet the psychiatric needs caused by disasters amounts to destigmatization, albeit circumscribed, for both the consumers and providers. Intervention at the earliest onset of symptoms is cost-effective: prompt attention to any pathological sign portends untold benefits over time.

Yet many who are not victims of natural disaster find themselves temporarily homeless because of failure to recognize psychiatric symptoms and to seek treatment soon enough to avoid major disruption in their living situations. These persons may have behaved in such an aberrant fashion that they made continuation of their residency untenable. In the ensuing crisis they are brought for emergency psychiatric treatment either by alternately caring and exasperated family or by law officers. At that point, the easiest alternatives for placement are hospital or jail; both meet the immediate needs of domicile and treatment.

A child or youth, for example, may present at a hospital with various complaints that compel psychiatric evaluation. The patient turns out to be the victim of incest. The exposure of this history frequently prevents the victim's return home due to fear of expulsion or retaliation. Temporary hospital admission is the most expedient solution. The perpetrator of sexual abuse may also emerge from the crisis bereft of home and in need of psychiatric treatment. Incarceration becomes the route for care. Although functional and indicative of public concern, such placements are far from desirable.

Psychiatric crises often erupt when the family system "can't stand it anymore." "It,"—the deviant, the nonproductive, the senile, the abuser—is targeted for expulsion. When "it" cooperates with the treatment or rehabilitation urged by the family, the chances are good that "it" will be reintegrated into the family system, healthier for the process. An alternative positive outcome is that "it" leaves the complaining system in an orderly, supported way to begin life's next task.

The temporarily homeless in need of psychiatric care can rally support effectively so that placement will seldom be an unanticipated, taxing problem. We have come to expect publicly funded programs to mitigate the emotional chaos of being temporarily homeless.

THE EPISODICALLY HOMELESS

A number of individuals and families out there are just barely surviving. Their emotional and economic stability is precariously balanced. The constant demands of a family member with chronic, perhaps debilitating, illness is suffocating. Unhappy marriages propel partners to acts of desperation. It is not surprising, therefore, when these so-called marginal families, beset with myriad problems, who have perhaps fewer internal and certainly fewer external resources, become episodically homeless. Placement for such persons is seldom easy. These are victims of the "shoulds": they should have been born smarter, saved money for a rainy day, paid the insurance premium, gone to the marriage counselor, not reverted to heavy drinking, chosen the secure job, never left those children unattended, obeyed the law, stopped at the traffic light, taken their medicine. Although our society channels help to these unfortunates, its delivery is designed to imply castigation for the failure to be self-sustaining. This message is internalized and experienced as "I'm definitely not okay."

At each shift from home to shelter or from a familiar shelter to an unfamiliar shelter, the self-respect of the homeless tends to become more fragile. Each time public assistance is sought, a challenge is posed to the self.[3] Very few money brokers, whether charitable trusts, banks, or governmental units, extend funds or credit without obtaining and verifying voluminous data: What do you want or need? Why? Where else have you applied? Who is involved? How do you propose to meet the conditions for continuing the proposed contract? For the upwardly mobile, such questions, though tedious and perhaps anxiety producing, are an opportunity to accentuate accomplishments. For the marginal applicant, such intrusiveness is not so benign. Recounting the events that led the person to make the application frequently becomes an emotional experience during which intra- and interpersonal conflicts expose recurring disappointments and failures.

Consider the generous grandmother who lives in government-subsidized housing and extends hospice to a grandchild, Jack, recovering from his first mental breakdown. A twenty-year-old high school graduate, Jack was self-supporting and sharing a furnished apartment with friends when he required hospital admission for treatment of his first psychotic episode. He responded well to treatment, with the expectation of progressive recovery. But upon discharge, Jack prefers not to participate in discharge planning. Mother and stepfather will not shelter him because he refuses follow-up treatment. Jack is not allowed to return to work without a medical release and loses his job. Jack's friends reject and evict him because he cannot keep up his share of the apartment. Jack seeks temporary shelter at his grandmother's. The housing authority warns grandmother that she is in violation of her contract and subject to eviction. Jack refuses to seek alternate housing. Grandmother's high blood pressure and diabetes get out of control and she develops symptoms of anxiety. She is referred to the psychiatric clinic.

Jack's psychotic symptoms return, but he refuses to seek treatment. Once he slaps grandmother and pulls the telephone out from the wall. Another time he threatens the neighbors. The family tries to get Jack treated against his will but cannot demonstrate that he is an immediate danger to himself or others. Upon learning that his family considers him "crazy," Jack hitchhikes to his natural father's home in another state.

Father has no available funds to assist Jack; Jack now qualifies for help only at a mission-type shelter. Unable to conform to mission rules, Jack must seek psychiatric attention or leave. At public expense, Jack is rehospitalized, accepts patienthood, complies with the treatment regimen, and recovery proceeds. Upon discharge, Jack agrees to placement in a halfway house and to social and vocational rehabilitation plans.

Jack becomes homeless only episodically, usually when he feels so well that he discontinues medicine and decompensates. The hospitalization cycle is repeated.

What happens to grandmother? As a result of the disruption Jack created, she is evicted from the housing project. With her health problems out of control and no one to care for her, she is temporarily placed in a nursing home where she lingers until her death. The family blames Jack for this regrettable course, which Jack learns about from a social worker who seeks to reconcile Jack with his family. Jack, however, feels the sting of guilt and rejection. For many years—perhaps forever—Jack will not initiate any contact with his family.

Now consider Jane. Jane, the apple of her father's eye, marries a fiscally irresponsible young man, Joe, who beats her. She soon requires medical and psychiatric treatment. Joe abandons her. Without funds, she asks father to foot the bill for this treatment and for separate housing. Father provides unstintingly. Joe returns. Jane forgives and promises to forego psychotherapy, and they try to make a go of the marriage. When this fails, Jane somehow finds her way into a religious cult that assumes total responsibility for her life. Disillusioned after a time, she leaves the cult and is again rescued from episodic homelessness by her father. Many times in her life she will be rescued by family, cults, women's shelters, perhaps hospitals. The public, however, takes little notice until her siblings put a stop to father's financial generosity. (Why should Jane run through father's money? What will father do when it's all gone? What right does Jane have to take their fair share of the inheritance?) Then Jane is thrown upon the public for the episodic "fix."

THE CHRONICALLY HOMELESS MENTALLY ILL

The desirability of having a home is unquestioned. Our very humanity may rest on having developed a homebase for cooperative, civilizing efforts.

> A homebase would permit older or infirm members of the group to stay behind and wait for the others to come back with food. "It is the home base," wrote Sherwood L. Washburn, a physical anthropologist at the University of California at Berkeley, "that changes sprained ankles and fevers from fatal diseases to minor ailments."[4]

Being homeless has long given rise to behaviors considered pathological in psychiatric circles. Consider Medea when her husband, the ambitious king of Corinth, banished her in order to take a more politically attractive wife; fearing the worst for her children, having no homebase to which to return, Medea slew her children and herself in a fit of rage. Scottish villagers, displaced during the Industrial Revolution, sought medical treatment for a condition diagnosed as "chronic unremitting nostalgia, simple or complex."[5]

By the mid-twentieth century mental patients could be restrained with major tranquilizers. It was the first step toward deinstitutionalization, the policy of discharging psychiatric patients from large, long-term hospitals as soon as possible into the community, with a plan for outpatient follow-up treatment.

But discharge *where* exactly? With no receiving family or income to meet basic needs, most mental patients become permanently institutionalized, never to be functional on the outside. Nonetheless, in 1975 the *Dixon* vs. *Weinberger* decision (1) set out the guideline of "least restrictive" level of care/setting as an integral part of treatment, (2) declared unnecessary institutionalization, considered to be the most restrictive setting, debilitating, and (3) mandated the government to fund alternatives to hospitalization.

Not everyone interprets deinstitutionalization as a positive government policy. Andrew Scull has written:

> . . . many negative rights given to mental patients in recent years
> have as their primary function the enabling [of] the state to disguise
> neglect as humane concern for the rights of the deviant . . . until
> 1950 . . . [it was] simply less expensive . . . to store "social junk"
> in "monasteries for the mad" than . . . create extensive support
> services necessary to sustain them in the community . . . now . . .
> rights are compatible with the overriding need of the state to pro-
> cess "nonproductive" citizens in the cheapest way possible.[6]

It is now commonly recognized that inadequate treatment facilities have been provided in local areas. In fact, the metropolitan media have flooded the public with relevant information. The needs of the homeless mentally ill have become a popular cause with mental health professionals and concerned citizen advocates.

Many of the mentally ill homeless are not just mentally ill. They are also epileptic, diabetic, blind, or deaf. Many stutter. Others abuse alcohol as well as drugs. Psychometric studies reveal that some are mentally retarded, some are brilliant. Many are sexually promiscuous, while others eschew all interpersonal contact. These individuals would benefit from placement, where staff could deal with the complexities of their multiple major diagnoses. Yet these patients are often excluded from placement precisely because they have multiple health and emotional problems.

Consider the situation of Lorenzo. Lorenzo is still a relatively young man who retains some of his good looks even when stooped with cold and lost in fantasy. He never graduated from high school or developed much of a trade. His older, middle-class mother doted on her only child and, seeking advantage for him, set him apart from other children in the working-class neighborhood. His alcoholic father shared his semi-skilled trade and his liquor with Lorenzo.

While still in his early teens, Lorenzo was removed from his home as a result of multiple family problems, rage reactions, and petty crimes. In a major fracas at the boy's home he sustained injuries with lasting neurological insult. Subsequently his behavior presented even more of a management problem, and so he was brought for psychiatric attention.

In his late teens, under medication, Lorenzo returned to the parental home. But he soon found he was ill prepared to achieve the lifestyle he wanted: money to spend on girls, liquor, stylish clothes, a sports car, a stereo—"the works." His mother tried to keep him from his "low-life" friends. Violent conflict often resulted. He attacked his mother, his father for abusing the mother, and neighbors when he thought they were spying on him.

Lorenzo, not unlike his peers, used street drugs, hustled a buck any way he could, engaged in petty crime, and, after many brushes with the law, was imprisoned. Though he had been noncompliant with psychiatric treatment while at home, in prison, the epitome of a maximally structured environment, he stopped using street drugs and was treated with psychotropics with impressive success. Upon release he moved into housing arranged by, but apart from, his mother. But without structure and encouragement, Lorenzo was evicted and brought to the hospital. His faddish clothing attracted more attention than his veiled thought disorder. He was refused admission; the staff thought all he needed was a place to stay.

His most recent landlord apologetically refused to take him back because "Lorenzo starts talking with those devils in the commode. He's pulled it out from the wall twice and flooded the house. And I just can't afford to replace the carpet again." Fearing robbery and assault, Lorenzo was afraid to return to the mission-type shelter. He could not be housed in a facility for the mentally ill because he was neither stabilized on psychotropics nor actively involved in a treatment and rehabilitation program. The drug rehabilitation center refused to admit him because no clients who required psychotropic medication were accepted.

Lorenzo lived on the streets and in the hospital. His mother would send a few dollars by friends as often as she could. Carefully avoiding authorities, he would hustle hospital visitors and sneak remaining food from hospital trays. He occasionally found a rescuer and disappeared.

Periodically, Lorenzo's behavior would be dominated by persecutory hallucinations; he would be hospitalized briefly in the general hospital, longer in the state hospital. He always benefited from a structured setting and medication but would be released to virtually the same vacuum of social supports. Lorenzo valued his freedom to refuse placement, but he would say "sometimes things are so bad out there, they just despair you to another dimension."

After years of his mother's determined struggle with the Social Security Administration, Lorenzo now has regular income (Social Security Disability based on his parents' earnings) and Medicare. The mother's health is deteriorating. The father died of pneumonia while he was hospitalized for treatment of injuries perpetrated by Lorenzo. Barely thirty years old, Lorenzo is now in the state mental hospital, where he is being treated for liver disease and his psychiatric problems. He does not yet qualify for nursing home placement nor, with his history, is he a candidate for a "less restrictive level of care."

In other circumstances Lorenzo's situation might have been easily corrected. We can readily imagine that family therapy at some point would have been beneficial. The mother's goals for her child to excel, to have a better life than other children in a high-crime neighborhood, are not unusual in themselves. These are, in fact, quite consistent with our society's goals of doing the best we can for our children. Consider Lorenzo's normal drives, not the least of which was to *be* normal in his development, particularly during adolescence. The task of developing his own identity was normal and necessary. His relationship to his peers, where their approval was more important than his parents', was normal. His evolving sexual drives were certainly within the normal range. The message of society to "go for it," to seek the things that he saw other teenagers getting, social acceptance through recreational use of street drugs, the desire for stereos, for fast cars or girlfriends, all of these are normal and are not necessarily shut down merely because at an early age Lorenzo appeared to have psychiatric problems.

The temptation to play the "if only" game is great: if only there had been family therapy, if only the schools could have met his educational requirements, if only he had had neighborhood peers with interests other than street life, if only his parents hadn't been fighting. But the "if only" game is a waste at the point at which Lorenzo is homeless. Where can he find bed and board, perhaps privacy, an opportunity to pursue rehabilitation?

In Lorenzo's frankly psychotic state, hospitalization was available to him, but when he improved on medication, he was soon placed in the least restrictive level of care. It might have been easy to place a man like this when he was young and appealing, and hope that he would stay forever. But this is rarely the case: a young man is seldom able to shut out society's messages to try again. There is the great hope that whatever was wrong was temporary, and the patient discontinues the medications when he feels better. The medical model would term these periods of remission; but under slight stress and without an adequate support system, the patient frequently bounces back, either to the hospital or to the housing agency for another placement.

Agency staff hardly veil their anger at such patients. They are usually direct and punitive. Some agencies have a policy not to *re*place patients who thwart an agency plan. The message to the patient is clear: "If you can't abide by our rules and take our recommendations on our terms, then do the best you can on your own. Get somebody else to try to help you. Don't come back here." The patient perceives this as "you don't want to help me."

What these agencies offer such patients has little variety. Shelters or boarding houses usually have rules that help operators achieve order, but are inconvenient for the residents. Overcrowding obviates the possibility of any privacy for sleep, use of toilet facilities, retreat, reflection, rest, or pursuit of personal relationships, particularly sexual relationships. No attention is given to individual needs. The norms of such institutions give conflicting messages to patients. Words encourage responsibility for one's self, one's behavior, one's medical care. Yet the rules about hours and guests, the lack of variety in diet, and the staff control of one's medication debilitate and often infantilize patients. It is all done, nevertheless, in the spirit of caring for the patient's needs.

While society has organized many ways for young people to mediate adolescent separation from the primary family, all these possibilities are closed for the young person who is chronically mentally ill. The message is clear: despite the fact that you have no outward signs of illness and society constantly wonders "what's the matter with you?" "why can't you work all the time?" "why are you here?," there is no hope for you.

The Lorenzos have questions, too. To a certain extent, they rebel and go through years of testing and trying and searching. One of the truly great difficulties for such young men is to be urged to accept the limitations of patienthood, to be placed in housing with people unlike themselves in age and primary disability or general circumstances, to adjust their goals downward, to accept that their lives will be greatly different from the lives of others.

Concurrently, however, patients are told, "Despite the fact that you most probably will never be what you had aspired to be at one time, or what your parents hoped for you at one time, or what your school tests indicated you had the capacity to become at one time, you are able to do *some* kind of work.'' This message is as confusing for mental health workers as it is for patients. In response to the need for housing and shelter, one must always be cognizant of young chronic patients' fluctuating states of consciousness, where they are in their development, and how their needs might be inconsistent with the state's. Any other response frustrates patients and alienates them from the very system that attempts to assist during this time.

The Lorenzos have problems with the health care system when they develop physical problems. Psychiatric patients have particular difficulty obtaining treatment for ordinary health needs. Normal aches and pains are not dealt with normally, even when patients are in a stage of reasonable remission, reporting the complaint based on accurate perceptions. Their complaints are frequently questioned, challenged, derided, and sometimes even dismissed. After all, they are ''just psych patients.'' The patients are acutely aware of how their histories of psychiatric diagnoses affect staff's reluctance to attend to complaints if they are other than psychiatric. Many patients refuse to go for care of broken arms or painful ingrown toenails or psoriasis because of the response they receive from the helping facility.

Some patients do not develop mental illness until midlife, particularly those diagnosed as manic depressive. Frequently these patients have been high achievers or have at least conformed with society's expectations of them at previous levels of development.

Consider the example of Sue, now in her mid-forties. Her symptoms developed when she was in her late thirties. She had four children between the ages of seventeen and twenty-three when she was abandoned by her husband. She was never able to assume the head-of-the-household parental role. Although she had been a successful suburban housewife, Sue had no education that would support a career outside the home and was unable to maintain the standard of living afforded by her ex-husband. The children needed parental support and guidance, and rather than assuming the caretaking responsibility for Sue, they elected to reside with their father. This eroded Sue's self-confidence even more. Perhaps it also took away motivation to recover. Unable to accept the quality of care available in the public sector, she was forced back into a dependent role on her ailing, elderly mother, an arrangement much resented by Sue's brother for its deleterious effects on the mother's health.

This patient gradually became restless and rebellious in the confines of her mother's household. She left for the streets, where she could forget the pain of rejection by her children and husband and seek satisfaction of her normal needs to be reaffirmed as a person and as a female. Ultimately, she chose the life of a prostitute, preferring the mercy of the unknown over whatever her mother or the community might have been able to offer.

Occasionally when she ran afoul of the law, principally because of her loud and unladylike behavior, uncontrolled during lapses of medication, she was brought to the hospital, "tuned up" to some extent, and returned to her preferred lifestyle. Over the years her appearance continued to change, not just by the normal hazards of aging, but by inadequate facilities for personal hygiene, lack of attention to overall grooming, poor diet, and a cultivated indifference to her person.

In the meantime Sue had solved her housing needs by working as a prostitute. Moderately obese in ill-fitting garb, dirty, with stringy, unkempt hair, always with a suspicious or scowling mien, ever ready to respond to intentional or accidental slights, she earned little. She discontinued her psychiatric medications. She was dependent on the largesse of "down-and-outers" a block away from skid row. Though she had taken her fate into her own hands, she was so disorganized that she did not have the paraphernalia to qualify as a bag lady.

Sue was periodically brought from the jail to the hospital for psychiatric treatment and occasionally would agree to remain for several weeks. She obtained a good remission with medicine and care: she departed with her thinking as "clear as a bell," talking "like a Republican." Her family—near-invalid mother now older, siblings totally occupied trying to meet their own families' needs, young adult children struggling with their own age-appropriate tasks—has shut its various doors as well as unlisted all telephone numbers. Upon discharge, Sue insisted on depending solely on her own wits and enterprise. It remains unknown whether or not she desires to attempt "regular" routine work again. Professional assessment of her ability to obtain and maintain such work is irrelevant because Sue does not seek advice or counsel.

In her county she is eligible for free outpatient treatment for psychiatric problems, thyroid dysfunction, and other diseases—especially sexually transmitted ones. Little realistic hope inspires the caregivers that Sue will avail herself of the help available. Her behavior patterns foster compassionate understanding of the rejecting family. Indeed, the caregivers find great difficulty in sustaining their professional roles—tax supported, publicly sanctioned—without punitive attitudes. It is difficult to help someone who does not want to be helped within the prescribed guidelines.

Mental health professionals look for every shred of potential to link patients with their families, to facilitate the reestablishment of bearable bonds. This work—even when fruitless—is always poignant. The police bring these people to the hospital, sometimes unidentified, naked or smartly dressed, hoarse after attempting to direct traffic, almost crippled from blisters on the feet, bruised from the rescue from the ledge where they had been poised to leap, confused, distraught, yet rarely amnesic.

Such a patient is Andrew, a heavily bearded young man, malnourished, his feet showing much abuse from weeks of walking. He invites incredulity as he reluctantly gives his history bit by bit. But, yes, it is true that he earned a masters degree in music performance a few years ago. His mother will come for him again if he wishes, although his father, a highly successful pathologist, cannot take time to make another trip. The family has been able to maintain private medical insurance for Andrew. After a brief hospital admission with some improvement, he vanishes again into the streets and shelters, certainly unwilling, perhaps unable, to try social rehabilitation again.

Another example is Bridget, almost eighteen, admitted to the hospital because she has attempted suicide again. She has not been living with her parents for several years. Her family's lack of concern is perplexing. Her mother, a war bride, speaks little English: she spends most of her time caring for a totally disabled twenty-year-old child. The father, hard working, is a long-distance trucker. Older siblings and uncles and aunts have done their stint. Bridget, a victim of incest, has gone from relative to hospital to "placement" to streets since she was fourteen. Her perception is accurate: there is no home for her.

Letters tell the helping professionals why parents can no longer allow the patient to remain at home. Their doctors advise them that their health cannot tolerate the strain of having the unpredictable patient around. The patient burned the house down and now there is no room in the apartment. The patient is demanding and uncooperative. The patient's moods are worrisome and have erupted into violence before. Rarely is there a story where the patient is expelled after only one episode of uncontrollable destruction or violence. There have usually been several attempts at reintegration into the home or at least with some part of the extended family. Professionals try to convince the family that the patient can accept some responsibility for comportment, that each party has rights to set behavioral limits in the interest of safety and integrity. Home is promoted as a place where rules of behavior exist and one chooses whether or not to abide by them or to enforce them. When the modern family can adopt this legalism wholeheartedly, rehabilitation of the difficult, otherwise homeless, patient proceeds with reasonable hope of success.

Some of these sketches suggest that the homeless had much opportunity in their families of origin. What are the histories of the mentally ill who were born into poverty? In homes and communities where disability and deprivation are common, a greater tolerance for deviance seems to prevail. Life's vicissitudes are accepted with more equanimity: not every problem requires a solution. Illness and affliction may be accepted as having great meaning: a test of faith for the caretakers, a punishment for riotous living, a force outside the victim seeking to do harm. Very seldom will the families see the patient's patienthood as something over which to exercise control.

The poor family is generally very protective and concerned, and it is here that the ravages of mental illness wreak the gravest harm. One must question the wisdom of maintaining the ill family member. Such a patient may monopolize emotional resources within the family unit, bring social ostracism on the children, precipitate crises that drive others out of the home prematurely and sometimes even require a wage earner to give up employment in order to give care. In the world of poverty there is never enough of anything—food, clothing, space, recreation, privacy, cigarettes, bedclothing, options for change, sometimes even hope that life can improve.

MEETING THE NEEDS OF THE HOMELESS MENTALLY ILL

Housing needs vary for each individual, depending on the nature of the illness, the patient's age and stage of life, previous lifestyle, religious preference, gender, and identity. When there are choices, homogeneity will attract and hold patients simply because the level of comfort is more specific. Youth need the possibility for adventure. The elderly need peace and quiet, with social stimulation nonetheless. Paranoid patients need adequate privacy to retreat from the environment when stresses begin to build. The depressed need constant companionship available. Most people need privacy to pursue intimate relationships. The transient mentally ill need primarily the opportunity to bathe, to launder clothing, to eat simple food, and to have shelter made available without having to "spill one's guts" as the price.

Until inspired solutions are developed, basic shelter and housing must be provided. For the homeless mentally ill, how should it be financed? In order for consistent, decent standards to prevail, the federal government must take leadership responsibility on a broad scale, if not for the total plan. Ideally, such a plan should be adapted to the individual's stage of development within the course of the diagnosed illness.

Physicians should take the mentally ill patient's complaints seriously and never dismiss them as imaginary or exaggerated. Trusting relationships enhance the likelihood of effective care.

Obviously, it would be desirable for the patient to attend the same outpatient clinic regularly so that medication can be titrated specifically, taking into account subtleties of thought, mood, and behavior changes. The patient needs to accept the responsibility to report any changes in function rather than adopting the passive role of withholding information unless specifically asked.

Medication is always an issue for the chronically ill patient because when one maintains improvement for a period of time there is the temptation to stop taking it. But for the homeless, where adjustment is tenuous at best, this is a treacherous route. Many shelters, missions, and boarding homes insist on keeping and dispensing medicine. This accomplishes the obvious but serves to infantilize patients. Yet it is very difficult to expect these patients to take medicines as prescribed without monitoring. Compliance is enhanced when any medicine can be taken once—or twice at most—a day; this weakens the message that every problem can be solved with a pill, and patients can pursue employment with less stigma or inconvenience.

Should patients work for their benefits? In our society, where the work ethic is so pervasive and production so valued, participation at some level in community chores is usually therapeutic and essential for self-esteem. Wages for work have merit as a method of reintegrating patients into normalcy.

Vocational rehabilitation planners have devised functional and attractive work patterns that accommodate the vagaries of the mentally ill. These are underutilized and underexplored. The public is mystified by the appearance of the unemployed mentally ill: "everybody has problems: but they work." It is hard to understand that the symptoms of the invisible handicap are alienation and decreased motivation. The manifest symptoms of disorganization and violence arouse distrust, anxiety, and ultimately rejection in many potential employers.

Most citizens appreciate the present state of the national economy. We will tax ourselves to help those who are less able to help themselves. Individuals in churches and agencies have stepped forward to answer such needs. Ingenious networking, volunteers extending their energies, churches opening their doors, domiciles adding mattresses and cots—all are measures of creative, sacrificial effort mounted in the private sector. More of the same is needed.

REFERENCES

1. Cordes C. The plight of homeless mentally ill. Monitor (American Psychological Assn). 1984; 15(2):1–13.
2. U.S., National Institutes of Health. Disaster assistance for crisis counseling and training. Grant to Harris County MHMRA. January 6, 1984.
3. Segal SP, Spocht H. A poor house in California, 1983: oddity or prelude? J Natl Assoc Soc Workers. 1983; 28:319–23.
4. Boyce R. What made humans human? New York Times Magazine. April 8, 1984:80–95.
5. Cullen G. Nosologia methodica. Edinburgh: J. Carfrae, 1820.
6. Scull A. In: Psychiatric patient rights and patient advocacy: issues and evidence. Human Science Press, Community Psychology Series. 1982; 7:266.

PART IV

ORGANIZATION OF HEALTH CARE SERVICES

16

Access to Care

Alexander Elvy

Health care, especially continuous, comprehensive primary care, remains beyond the reach of the homeless throughout this country. It would be unfair, however, to say that the homeless are completely out of touch with the health care system or that they never have an opportunity to be treated by a physician or other health professional. In fact, they do come in contact with organized medicine—albeit under less than desirable circumstances in most instances. The homeless person's contact with the health care system generally takes place in a county or municipal hospital emergency room,[1,2] and only when traumatic or life-threatening circumstances force them to seek medical attention. As a result, the health care the homeless receive is crisis oriented, fragmented, limited, and of questionable long-term value. In effect, it is health care that is at best minimal.

That the homeless are in dire need of comprehensive medical care is an undisputed fact; their multiple and complex medical problems are well described throughout this text. That their medical needs are as yet unmet is also undisputed.

HEALTH CARE AND THE HOMELESS:
A LIMITATION

In discussing the specific health care needs of the homeless, an important limitation must be mentioned: very little hard data or literature is available that speaks to this issue. However, much information is available on the characteristics of low-income groups and the poor and on their impact on the health care systems throughout the country. The homeless and the poor have much in common, although two circumstances differentiate the groups: first, the homeless are, by definition, without shelter; and second, they suffer a higher incidence of psychiatric illness than is generally found among low-income groups.

ACCESS TO CARE

Now, many an advocate who has analyzed the health care needs of the homeless is quick to point to the wide chasm between the homeless and their access to traditional medicine. While it is true that most medical institutions have been unable, and at times unwilling, to reach out to the homeless, to cite this as the only reason the homeless remain outside the scope of traditional medicine is to ignore the complexity of the problem. In broad terms, there appear to be three major reasons why the homeless have difficulty obtaining medical care:

1. The health care system itself: the manner in which health care is traditionally delivered in this country.
2. Special needs of the homeless: the unique nature of the homeless person and homelessness itself.
3. Attitudes of health professionals: values generally held by health care providers toward the homeless patient that inhibit care, even when the patient can pay with Medicaid, for example.

ORGANIZED MEDICINE AND
THE HOMELESS

Given the financial, psychological, political, cultural, and professional context of private-practice medicine, it is safe to say that there are few physicians who see homeless people in their private offices. The homeless sometimes receive treatment from a physician who donates time and skill to a shelter clinic, such as the Zacchaeus Clinic in Washington, DC (see Chapter 24). But even this is a rather limited option for the population, since not many such clinics exist.

Too often, the only medical care available to the homeless is offered in a hospital setting at a county or municipal institution financed by tax levy funds.[3-7] But even under the best of circumstances, interaction with traditional medical institutions is a frustrating, overwhelming experience for the vast majority of the homeless. Confronted with myriad protocols and procedures of conventional hospital medicine, most homeless people would rather do without medical care than subject themselves to such an ordeal.

By far the major barrier to receiving hospital care is financial. Fees for an outpatient visit at a public or voluntary hospital in New York City, for example, can range from under $20 to well over $100 per visit for patients without medical coverage. The issue is simple: Institutional policies that require payment prior to treatment make emergency room care, clinic visits, and inpatient care largely unavailable to the homeless. This is especially true at not-for-profit, voluntary hospitals, which are under ever increasing pressure to minimize their operating deficits.[8,9] And while most municipal hospitals will allow a patient to be seen in the emergency room or clinic irrespective of his or her ability to pay (a factor which largely accounts for the significant deficit with which most municipal hospitals are strapped),[3,4,6] the nonpaying patient is rarely received with enthusiasm or unqualified acceptance. All nonpaying patients are billed and dunning letters sent to delinquent patients, making many fearful and reluctant to return for follow-up care.

Of course, Medicaid has done much to provide coverage to the vast majority of the low-income population. Yet many of the homeless remain outside of the safety net provided by such coverage.[10-13] Many people working with the homeless cite repeated instances of their clients' inability to secure Medicaid and other entitlements, such as public assistance and Supplemental Social Security (SSI).

In order for people to receive Medicaid, for example, two major obstacles must be overcome. People must have both a stable address and "proper documentation." In regard to the latter, as part of the normal application process for Medicaid in New York City an applicant is required to provide the following:

1. Identification
2. Current or past residence
3. Citizenship
4. Social Security card

5. Indication of disability, if any
6. Indication of previous support by family or friends
7. Past employment record
8. Current income and financial resources, if any[14]

Few homeless people carry such detailed documents with them. Since they rarely have a safe place to store anything, requests for one or more documents virtually guarantees noncompliance. And securing these documents is nearly impossible for the homeless, who are generally estranged from their families and out of touch with agencies that replace such documents once they are lost or misplaced. Thus, the documentation required by entitlement programs virtually eliminates the homeless from adequate coverage, unless they are aggressively assisted by someone who helps them get the needed papers or who can have some of the standard documentation requirements waived. Additionally, criteria for Medicaid eligibility vary widely from state to state;[11,15] and some states do not even allow homeless people to secure Medicaid or public assistance, even if they can pass the means test. For example, during a visit to the Pine Street Inn in Boston, in the fall of 1983, staff from St. Vincent's were told that homeless persons staying in any shelter in Massachusetts were automatically ineligible for public assistance or Medicaid. And beyond Medicaid, programs such as Hill-Burton, which mandates a hospital to provide free care for the medically indigent in exchange for government subsidies for their building plants, have proven to be failures in addressing the health needs of this population.[16]

Organizational procedures and the standard practices of medical institutions also provide formidable barriers to the homeless when they seek care for their afflictions. Without a doubt, proper documentation of the patient's visit to the facility is crucial in order to protect the legal rights of the patient, the physicians, and the medical complex. Registration forms, clinic cards, referral sheets, lab slips, and charts are among the standard forms demanded by all medical institutions; without them, sound medical care would be virtually impossible to provide. But, matters that are simple to most of us—completing a registration form, having one's clinic card readily available at each visit, or giving the physician a detailed medical history—become difficult obstacles for the homeless patient to negotiate. As a homeless woman recently told me, "I just come here for the doctor to look at my eyes. What does that have to do with where I was born or my mother's name before she got married?"

For many, being guarded about the past insures a degree of anonymity that they hope will decrease potentially negative consequences. And medical staff can never be certain how accurate the information given by the homeless person is, particularly the histories of those afflicted with past and present psychiatric illness. So, unfortunately, many patients refuse medical care rather than give the most minimal history.

Another equally significant barrier is the manner in which health care is dispensed at most hospitals. Going from the emergency room to the primary care clinic; to the lab for blood work, urine analysis, x-rays; to the specialty clinic; then back to the primary care clinic can be overwhelmingly confusing to the homeless person. One homeless woman, who was seen by three or four different doctors for her multiple medical problems without understanding who had primary responsibility for her medical care, described this to me as a form of harassment that she could do without.

Keeping follow-up appointments and complying with medical protocols also decreases the odds against continuous, comprehensive care. Life on the streets or movement from shelter to shelter implies a life of massive disorganization. Without structure, one day merges into the next. The homeless are frequently heard asking, "What day is it?" "Has the weekend come yet?" Poor time orientation is not only a problem for follow-up clinic visits, but also for proper medication compliance; that is, if the medication has not gotten wet or been lost or stolen.

Lack of outreach to the target population by traditional medical institutions also creates obstructions.[5,17-19] To treat the homeless, it is imperative that medical professionals get to "where they're at." The homeless rarely come to a medical facility unless they are seriously ill. Taking medicine to the homeless—bringing it to the shelter, to the street, or to the church basement or storefront—significantly increases the chances of reaching this population. Even if hospitals opened their doors to the homeless and removed every financial and procedural barrier possible, it is safe to say that the homeless would continue to stay away. Therefore, reaching out to this population is key.

Then there is the issue of transportation. Many programs throughout the country have been successful in setting up on-site shelter clinics, with backup medical facilities that provide more technical services when needed. However, availability of transportation to the backup facility is crucial to treatment compliance and high quality care.[5,20] All staff at St. Vincent's Hospital in New York who work with the homeless recognize that free transportation increases the likelihood that patients from the shelter will keep their follow-up medical appointment at the backup hospital site. One shelter we service is three blocks from the hospital;

still, some patients there have insisted that they be picked up as a condition for coming to the clinic.

HOMELESSNESS ITSELF AS PART OF THE PROBLEM

As a group, the homeless are enmeshed in a world of alienation and are often fragmented from conventional societal norms. Forced to exist on the fringes of society, their lives are fraught with trauma, uncertainty, and fear. While there is evidence that the homeless are not a homogeneous group and that there are some "higher functioning homeless," chronic street-dwellers are ill equipped to fend for themselves except in a minimal way, especially when the vast amount of psychiatric illness among the population is factored in.[21-23] Therefore, to ask homeless persons to seek ongoing health care on their own is to ignore the nature and effects of prolonged life on the streets.

For the homeless, health care is a luxury that follows the pressing need for hot meals, shelter from the elements, and an environment safe from predators. The homeless use low visibility as a survival mechanism. By fading into the background, they keep their fragile environments intact and feel safe. Medical examinations and other forms of care can be threatening to the homeless person. Many decline medical care in order to remain as invisible as possible.

To sum up, a homeless person's life is one of extreme instability. Any event can dramatically alter the fragile equilibrium. Therefore, it is absolutely essential that these factors be taken into consideration in the development of any medical program aimed at reaching this group.

MEDICAL CARE, "VALUES," AND THE TREATMENT OF THE HOMELESS

Beyond tangible barriers to care, the attitudes and values of health workers may equally limit effective treatment of the homeless. In discussing this phenomenon, E. Erkel has stated:[24]

> The majority of health professionals share similar ethnic [cultural] class values and life styles. [And] a distinct middle-class bias pervades the norms for health care consumers as a consequence of health professionals' social background and the phenomenon of ethnocentrism. Studies have shown (1) that health care providers prefer middle class consumers because of their mutual social char-

acteristics, i.e., educational and behavior patterns, and (2) that there is a tendency by health care providers to view lower-class consumers in terms of unfavorable stereotypes. Thus, public (lower-class) health care consumers are viewed less favorably than private (middle and upper class consumers). . . . Socially undesirable patients include alcoholics, the physically dirty, the uneducated and the very poor. The poor are disliked for their uncleanliness, noisiness and lack of cooperation and compliance. Public health nurses sometimes reject patients for care because they live in a "bad neighborhood or one with a high crime rate." Researchers . . . observed that providers volunteered remarks indicative of their perceptions of their patients' social status, including derogatory comments and indicative gestures.

Such attitudes can be damaging. In many instances, the homeless *are* physically unclean or infested with lice. This is to be expected. Living on the streets or moving from shelter to shelter provides scant opportunity to maintain personal hygiene. The homeless should not be punished for their circumstances by being denied needed medical care.

Care providers must be aware of imposing their feelings and attitudes onto the patient. Body language or facial expression that may be construed by the homeless patient as a form of disapproval or rejection of their lifestyle should be avoided. There is probably no quicker way to lose a homeless person's participation in the treatment process than to indicate to them that you are not pleased with the way they conduct their lives. However, opportunities for giving needed constructive advice are possible after a meaningful relationship between the homeless person and the care provider is established.

And what is important for the hands-on-care professional is equally important for the staff of the entire medical facility. The work of the outreach team makes little sense if it is aborted by an act of insensitivity on the part of someone in the emergency room or inpatient ward when the patient comes in contact with one of these services. If a medical facility is truly serious about providing care to the homeless, the entire facility must contribute to the effort. Directives should be sent from the highest administrative levels to all personnel indicating the commitment of the facility to the treatment of the homeless and the expectation that care will be provided to this population with respect and dignity.

INCREASING ACCESS TO CARE

While comprehensive, model medical programs are outlined in other chapters, minimal program requirements should include:

1. An on-site team to provide health care where the patients are—in shelters, temporary residences, storefronts.

2. A backup facility capable of providing a broad range of medical services:

   a. primary care clinics,
   b. emergency room services,
   c. subspecialty clinics,
   d. psychiatric services,
   e. inpatient care,
   f. ancillary testing, x-rays,
   g. pharmacy.

3. Provision of services to the homeless regardless of their ability to pay, while outreach staff explore all possibilities of reimbursement—Medicaid, Medicare, Hill–Burton funding, charity and free care, direct-targeted governmental funding, foundation support, and others.

4. Transportation to and from the core hospital facility.

5. Sensitivity training for staff in direct contact with the homeless population.

6. Appropriate personnel—social workers, aides—to manage the patients' interaction with the health care facility.

7. Overall institutional sanction for the program.

While the homeless are difficult to treat, they can be reached, but major adjustments must be made to tailor medical care to the particular characteristics of the patients. However, if a medical facility has the courage to develop a reasonable program geared toward eliminating traditional barriers, both concrete and intangible, increased access to medical care for the homeless patient can be assured.

REFERENCES

1. Brown RE. Poverty and health in the United States. Clin Pediatrics. 1969; 8:495–98.
2. Coleman AH. A social system to improve health care delivery to the poor. J Natl Med Assoc. 1969; 61:192–94.
3. Roman S. Public hospitals—there are no alternatives. Urban Health. 1979; 8:7.
4. Wolfe S, Goldman F, Richardson H. The fiscal crisis of New York City: the conflict in allocation of resources to the public and private health sectors. Consumer Health Perspectives. 1980; 6(7):1–6.

5. Bengnen L, Yerby A. Low income and barriers to use of health services. New Engl J Med. 1968; 278:541–46.
6. Brown R. Public hospitals on the brink: their problems and their options. J Health Politics, Policy & Law. 1983; 7:927–46.
7. Law R. Primary care and the poor in the inner cities of New York and Washington, USA. J Royal Coll Gen Practitioners. 1972; 22:679–93.
8. Sagen A. Why urban voluntary hospitals close. Health Services Research. 1983; 18:451–75.
9. Raynen G. Healthy profits. Health & Soc Services J. 1982; 92:1438–40.
10. Wilensky G, Berk ML. Health care, the poor, and the role of Medicaid. Health Affairs. 1982; 1:93–100.
11. Davis K, Gold M, Makuc D. Access to health care for the poor: does the gap remain? Ann Rev Pub Health. 1981; 1:159–82.
12. Wilensky G. Poor, sick and uninsured. Health Affairs. 1983; 2(2):91–95.
13. Gortmaker SL. Medicaid and the health care of children in poverty and near poverty. Med Care. 1981; 19:567–82.
14. Guide to documentation for the Medicaid application. New York City Office of Public Affairs Publication, Pub. No. W296C.
15. Davidson SM. Variations in state Medicaid program. J Health Politics, Policy and Law. 1978; 3:54–70.
16. New York hospitals not meeting Hill–Burton charity requirements (news item). Health Planning Manpower Report. 29 August 1979; 8:18.
17. Reaching the unreachables: Lincoln Hospital mental health services, Bronx, New York. Hosp & Comm Psych. 1968; 19:350–53.
18. Aday L. Economic and noneconomic barriers to the use of needed medical services. Medical Care. 1975; 13:447–56.
19. Bellen SS, Geiger HJ: The impact of a neighborhood health center on patients' behavior and attitudes relating to health. Medical Care. 1972; 10: 224–39.
20. Liberman A, Fougerousse J. Community-based outpatient clinic and transportation service. Hosp Topics. 1970; 48(4):70–80.
21. Homeless could use state hospitals, community shelters (news item). Clin Psych News. July 1982:35.
22. Many homeless need psychiatric help (news item). Psych News. March 1983:4.
23. Gershing J. Homeless in New York. New York: Pharos of Alpha Omega Honor Medical Society, 1983.
24. Erkel E. The implications of cultural conflict for health care. Health Values. 1980; 4:51–57.

17

Health Care Teams in Work with the Homeless

Marianne Savarese

Webster defines teamwork as joint action by a group of people, in which each person subordinates individual interests and opinions to enhance the unity and efficiency of the whole.

And there is the tale told by a Jewish sage:

> A man we know was given the unusual opportunity to take a guided tour of heaven and hell. In hell he found masses of pitiful creatures, starved and emaciated. Tables of delicious food were just within reach, but they were prohibited from eating because their outstretched arms were held rigid by long metal forks. They could not bend their elbows to feed themselves. In heaven, the setup was the same, but the people were happy, cheerful, healthy, and well-nourished. Our friend asked his guide to explain the difference. "Simple," he said. "In heaven they feed each other."[1]

The decision to utilize the team approach in giving health care to people who are homeless appears logical. A commitment to team development is crucial to that decision; without sustained focus on the team's developmental tasks, there will be no true teamwork.

THE EVOLUTION OF HEALTH TEAMS

As Dienst and Byl point out:

> Team approaches to health care have been developing steadily over
> the past 30 years in response to increasing concerns about the ac-
> cessibility, efficiency, and comprehensiveness of health care serv-
> ices. Concurrently, the growing interest in health maintenance . . .
> has drawn attention to the need for effective collaboration and co-
> operation among health professionals from different disciplines.[2]

Broad changes in health care trends have contributed to the evolution of the team approach. From a focus on treatment of disease, we
are now slowly moving toward a preventive approach.[1-5] As acute infectious illnesses were more easily cured, the incidence of chronic de-
generative diseases grew.[3,5] Changes in the health care system, such
as single physician to group practice, hospital-based care to community-
based care, and third-party payment for some forms of nonphysician
care, have increased opportunities to give services through teamwork.[5-7]
Other developments, such as improved education of the general public
and the entry of liberal, progressive persons into health care work, have
created a democratic, participatory environment for patients and health
professionals.[5]

> It is naive to bring together a highly diverse group of people and
> expect that, by calling them a team, they will in fact behave as a
> team. It is ironic indeed to realize that a football team spends 40
> hours a week practicing teamwork for the two hours on Sunday
> afternoon when their teamwork really counts. Teams in organiza-
> tions seldom spend two hours per year practicing when their ability
> to function as a team counts 40 hours per week.[7]

The use of teams in rendering primary health care programs has
become a familiar concept; this form of care for homeless people, however, is a new phenomenon. The homeless are a demographically diverse people with dissimilar health histories and varying individual
constitutional strengths. They share but one commonality—a lack of
housing. Homelessness creates physical and emotional consequences
that affect each homeless person in a variety of ways. If teamwork is
an effective way to provide comprehensive primary health care to meet
the needs of the general population,[4,8,9] then it is equally so for those
people who are homeless.

Before World War II general practitioners were widely used for primary health care.[4] During the 1940s, Dr. Martin Cherkasky utilized health care teams within the home care and family health demonstration projects at Montefiore Hospital in the Bronx.[7] In the 1960s, the Office of Economic Opportunity (OEO) funded the development of neighborhood health clinics, which were designed to remove barriers to health care for the poor by setting up clinics in their communities. These clinics utilized the interdisciplinary team approach and encouraged patients and community people to articulate their needs. The Martin Luther King, Jr., Health Center in New York City and the Institute for Health Team Development at Montefiore Hospital effectively combined the theory and practice of health teams during the early 1970s.[1,4,7,10,11]

The interdisciplinary team approach has been essential in caring for the frail elderly.[12] At St. Vincent's Hospital in New York, egalitarian teams are used to bring health care to the homebound elderly in the Chelsea Village Program,[1] which began in 1973 and is still in operation.

In this era of deep concern about costs of health services, dollars spent on health care are thoroughly scrutinized and not easily granted. Even though the rationale for the team lies in the need for coordination of care, "the ultimate survival of the team, as a mode for primary health care delivery, will depend on its ability to prove itself in the world of cost benefits and cost effectiveness."[5]

HEALTH TEAM DEFINED

Ducanis and Golin offer the following definition for a health team:

> An interdisciplinary team is a functioning unit composed of individuals with varied and specialized training who coordinate their activities to provide services to a client or group of clients. The team must recognize the principle that its specialist members need to become *one* functioning unit; just as the patient's life is *one* organismic whole.[10]

The health team is an entity. It is a corporate group of health providers whose separate and distinct skills are coordinated toward the common purpose of patient care, the accomplishment of which requires the interdependent and collaborative efforts of its members.[1,5,10,13-15] The health team is a compound, the elements of which are the various staff members.

The composition and size of the team should reflect the needs of the target population served, as well as the skills of the team members. There is a mutual dependence between team and patient. It is essential to remember that the patient is the reason for the team's existence.[1,5,10,11,14-16]

The members of this group must address certain developmental tasks to assure optimal team functioning. They must agree on common goals and priorities. This commonality of mission provides direction for the team and helps delineate its tasks. The specificity and clarity of goals, objectives, and priorities promotes ease of evaluation of achievements and outcomes.[1,5,7,10,11,13,15,17,18]

A democratic problem-solving approach must be utilized. Collaboration is the central element. When members agree on decisions and share in the decision-making process, commitment to the goal or task is heightened in each participant.[2,5,7,10,18]

Since teams are composed of human beings, a degree of conflict is inevitable, but its negative effects can be minimized. Each member's job must be clarified and understood. As conflicts arise relating to issues of territoriality, role negotiation through communication and conflict management must be employed. The clarification of role expectations among team members will help to minimize conflict during implementation of tasks and lead to achievement of goals.[2,3,5,7,10,11,13-15,17-20]

There must be ground rules that define how the team functions, norms that support the group's efforts. These are the unwritten rules that govern any group. They define acceptable and unacceptable behavior and therefore powerfully determine how members will behave. Repeated violation of norms often leads to psychological or physical expulsion. Flexible norms that encourage mutual support and open communication are essential for positive team energy and effectiveness.[7,10,18]

Recognition and concern for each member's personal and professional needs are important developmental tasks for the team. Respect for each one's professional ability helps to provide distinction when necessary. Encouragement and support of personal and professional development will ultimately enhance the team's growth.[1,3,7,13,15,18,21]

Leadership issues must be addressed. Leadership should be fluid, flexible, correlated to patient needs, and determined by the particular situation. All team members must be equally ready and willing to wield or yield authority.[1,3,5,7,11,13,18,19,22,23]

Ideally, membership should be stable. High turnover among members impedes the process of team maturation.[2,10,17] Members' personal and professional characteristics are important to an effectively functioning team: self-confidence, ability to give and receive criticism, tolerance and flexibility, a humanistic outlook and sensitivity to patient priorities, noncompetitiveness, being articulate and direct in communication, and most of all, a sense of humor.[1,13,16]

The most important developmental task of the team and a prerequisite for all other tasks is open communication. It is essential for goal setting, prioritizing of objectives, group decisions, role clarification, role negotiations, delegation of tasks, the show of mutual support and cohesiveness, and the emergence of leadership. It is essential that the team spend time promoting communication and addressing barriers to communication if team development and effective functioning are to be achieved.[1,4,7,8,10,12,13,15,17,19,20,22] Team meetings are a structured forum where case management as well as team maintenance issues can be discussed. The formality or informality of team meetings will be governed by the group's norms. Nevertheless, regular meetings held at intervals and times agreed upon by team members lead to effective communication. Meetings held *only* when conflicts arise lend a negative connotation to the meeting itself, which should instead be a welcomed event.[1,7,8,10,12,14,15,18,19,22] Charting is written communication essential for continuity of patient care. It is important to provide a common, accessible charting section where all professionals may enter their plans and impressions, as opposed to separate chart sections for each profession.[21,23] Perseverance may be necessary in order to provide an array of opportunities for open communication, verbal as well as written.

A HEALTH TEAM AT A NEW YORK SHELTER

Health care teams combining medicine, nursing and social work have traditionally been used within the primary care and outreach programs at St. Vincent's Hospital's Department of Community Medicine. Nutrition, psychiatry, health education, and oral surgery are available on a referral and consultative basis. The value of input from nonprofessional team members, such as bilingual clerk-receptionists and vehicle drivers, is recognized and utilized regularly.[14,23] When necessary, pharmacological input is sought from hospital or independent pharmacists. Although not part of the basic team, pharmacists' contributions are significant.[9,24] Medical, nursing, and social work students rotate through the programs and participate as team members for short periods of time.

The team approach has proven valuable in the delivery of primary care, efficiently addressing the complex needs of our diverse patient populations. The team approach also preserves the energy and stamina of its members through an atmosphere of mutual support and interdependence in the face of challenge.

For those people who are homeless, health care teams seem to be the ideal way to provide health care on-site at the shelters. Their health needs, as complex and diverse as those of the general population, are compounded by the homeless experience and all its inadequacies: shelter, food, clothing, hygiene, safety, and emotional support. Such needs cannot be met by one professional.

During a team approach workshop on health issues for the homeless, many of those present were members of shelter health teams. They commented on the value and necessity of the team approach:[15]

> Everyone here is working on a team and that can't be an accident. It has to have something to do with this population . . . you can't do this in private practice or alone.

> It's vital when you work with a population like the homeless, to be able to bounce off the team, what happened that day. . . . You are totally overwhelmed a lot of the time . . . it guards against burnout and keeps up the momentum that you need in this work.

> We found that it is impossible to work alone with this population. . . . It is impossible, mentally and physically, to deal with the numbers of people who approach you . . . so we adhere to the physical presence of the team members on site.

> We need the support of our team members . . . it's frustrating to work with this population . . . for the patient it shows a uniformity of approach from three, four or ten people on the team . . . it multiplies the effect of a congruent plan.

Accessibility to the health team is crucial for the homeless population, given their propensity toward isolation, suspicion, and dissaffiliation. Having a health team *on-site*, at the temporary residences of these men and women, helps to break down barriers to health care. In the program at St. Vincent's, physician–nurse–social worker teams are present at the shelters on a regular basis. In a manner analogous to home health care programs for the aged, these teams regularly visit the temporary living sites of the homeless. The consistent yet gentle persistence of a health team eventually can penetrate the homeless person's world. Team members must create a favorable milieu so that a trusting relationship may be established between the team and the patient. Such an atmosphere of acceptance helps the shelter residents to take the first step toward a health care system that is nonthreatening, accessible, and their own.

The team approach affords each patient a sense of control. They choose whether or not to approach the team, when to approach the team, and to whom, among team members, they will relate. Control over health care is a valuable possession that must be preserved in the men and women who have lost control over the other circumstances in their lives.

Victimized by a host of social, emotional, and economic ills, these people are often alienated from conventional institutions. One student observed: "Many of the psychiatric illnesses that I've seen in the homeless have as a consequence residual symptoms of social bluntedness and an intolerance to frustration. . . . People who cannot delay gratification or tolerate the frustration of a bureaucracy, will not seek medical or mental health experts on their own."[15] The health team is a positive representation of the health system to the homeless. At St. Vincent's, shelter health team members also staff hospital-based clinics established to meet the specific needs of the homeless. Such continuity strengthens the trusting relationship between patient and team and further facilitates the homeless person's access to traditional health care systems.

Since the needs of the homeless are so complex, a comprehensive approach to health care is vital. "For this population there is not just one problem that stands by itself. It is always interlocked with other problems, and you find that unless you attend to all of them together nothing is going to happen."[15] Through teamwork, patients are given access to a combination of professional skills that is greater than the sum of its parts. The comprehensiveness broadens as the shelter health team draws on the knowledge and skills of other professionals and nonprofessionals in consultation, and broadens further when extended teams are formed with shelter, hospital, or other agency staff members.

At a New York City shelter where we work, the health team was approached by Alice, a twenty-year-old woman, an unemployed high school graduate, recently estranged from her mother, with whom she had been living. She was in the early stages of pregnancy. Insolvent and without family and friends to rely on, she slept on the chairs of the shelter. She had the anger of an abandoned woman and the fears of an abandoned child. Her goals were to "get on welfare and keep my baby." As our team worked to meet the needs of this woman, we supported the developing maturity she showed in reaching out to us and at the same time exercised some control as she exhibited adolescent traits of manipulation and noncompliance.

After a physical examination at the shelter, our physician arranged prompt prenatal care for Alice. The nurse helped Alice integrate the information she received about nutrition, pregnancy, and childbirth. The social worker assisted Alice in securing public assistance and counseled her on issues relating to her pregnancy, future disposition of the baby, and her family relationships. The health team from the shelter communicated regularly with the OB/GYN staff at the hospital clinic and accompanied Alice to some of her clinic appointments. The shelter staff placed Alice in a lodging house run by the same organization that ran the shelter.

Thus Alice found a more appropriate home with a bed. She maintained regular contact with the health team at the shelter during the course of her pregnancy. Shelter staff helped her enter vocational training, since she planned to secure a job, find an apartment, and keep her baby. After she bore a healthy baby boy, she placed him in foster care, visited him on weekends, and returned to her training program while still living at the lodging home. The staff members who cared for her became her collective parents and close friends, and she showed us how proud she was of her baby and her progress toward reaching her original goals.

Six months later she reconciled with her mother, found an apartment in her mother's building, and began caring for her son in her own home each weekend. She would occasionally do volunteer work at the shelter and maintained contact with her case workers there.

"It is impossible to do this kind of work alone."[15] A team approach to health care is not only essential but is required to face the challenges presented by the target population. The team is not a haven that insulates its members against the overwhelming needs of the homeless. It is instead an operating network, an entity, that is optimally equipped to attend to such needs and that possesses an inherent support system that serves to diffuse the frustration felt and to replenish the energy spent by each team member.

THE RATIONALE FOR THE USE OF TEAMS

The health of human beings is affected by factors both within each person and in the environment. The effects of life stressors—poverty, unemployment, family alienation, crime, malnutrition, inadequate housing—in combination with acute and chronic disease are demanding of any health professional's skill. Deinstitutionalization of the chronically mentally ill has added more people poorly able to cope with life's problems to the pool of the population in need of health care.[25,26] One professional worker possesses neither the resources to address this complex array of interrelated health needs nor the ability to cope alone with such overwhelming societal atrocities. Through the team approach, we can attempt to address these complex problems with the combined skills and the mutual support of its members.[1,3-5,9-11,13,19,21,23,26,27] Health care can no longer be categorized by specialty or body system when the entire organism is in need. The health team must care for the patient as a holistic unit. Body and mind must not be separated.[1,4,10,15,28]

The team approach addresses a homeless patient's complex health problems historically, through comprehensive, continuous care. Continuity is especially crucial in the care of the chronically mentally ill, to ensure that services are available as needed to help them function adequately in the least restrictive setting.[4,25,26] The continuity of care rendered by a health team must possess the following characteristics:[25]

1. Longitudinality: consecutive, related episodes of care.
2. Individuality: care specific to the needs of the patient.
3. Comprehensiveness: a variety of services provided simultaneously to meet the patient's complex array of needs. Each service has its own temporal or longitudinal aspect.
4. Flexibility: flow of services changes as patients progress or decompensate.
5. Relationship and contacts: team members are interested in the patients and respond to them on a personal level.
6. Accessibility: free from barriers to service and the availability of an enabler who assists the patient through the system.
7. Communication: between patient and providers, and among all providers; the patient is assured of continuity and improved system efficiency.

Continuity of care may be achieved through teamwork. This concept minimizes turf problems among service providers and theoretically may be used with both medical and nonmedical treatment models. In fact, it effectively encourages a merging of treatment models: An interdisciplinary team is formed, for instance, when internists and psychiatrists work together, and the tendency of patients to split or to separate mind and body experiences is reduced.[4]

The team approach has its advantages and disadvantages. The team challenges many traditional norms:

1. Cooperation instead of competition
2. Group achievement instead of individual accomplishment
3. Cross-disciplinary sharing instead of unidisciplinary credit
4. Egalitarianism instead of authoritarianism
5. Consensual decisions instead of mandates
6. Flexibility instead of rigidity[2]

Establishing such norms and maintaining team effectiveness requires a conscious team effort.

The values of using a team approach, with shared responsibilities and frustrations, include psychological rewards that result in cohesiveness and mutual support.[1,7,15,17,18,23] For the patients, a team approach is valuable in that independence and control are encouraged, as they share in the health plan and decision making process.[10] The team members can enhance patients' understanding of their health problems and health plan, as well as their sense of trust, security, and control.[10,15] Finally, patients are less dependent on any *one* health professional.[10] They may choose to relate only to that person on the team with whom they most readily engage or to relate equally to all team members. Again, a sense of control is enhanced.

There are also disadvantages or drawbacks to the use of a team approach experienced by both the team members and the patients. When responsibilities and rewards are shared, the personal satisfaction of each professional is diminished.[10] "If team members fail to communicate and support each other, they will experience more anxiety which will drain team energy and spirit."[7] Issues of role misconceptions, overlap, and territoriality are also potential problems.[13,22] Breakdowns in communication lead to duplication of effort, fragmentation, forgotten or overlooked tasks, power struggles, competition, and resentments.[1,7,13,15,22] Strong professional identification and concerns about professional status are additional sources of conflict among team members.

Potential problems on the opposite end of the spectrum also occur in highly developed teams.[1,10,13,14,22] A highly cohesive team may avoid the true tasks of patient-centered care. A team maintenance focus may override a patient care focus and the team may be using its cohesiveness as a defense to avoid patient care issues.[5,10]

For patients, expectations of their increased involvement and independence, or the team's incongruous approach, may heighten their anxiety and confusion.[10] Patients may not be familiar with the concept of team health care, since they have been taught that the physician is primarily responsible for health care.[10,29]

The team approach may be exploited by a patient who is manipulative and intends to split the members of the team, pitting them against one another.

> L. E., a thirty-eight-year-old alcoholic man, was seen in the shelter clinic seventeen times over a period of eighteen months.
>
> Initially he requested medication because of insomnia. After referral to the consulting psychiatrist for treatment of anxiety and depression, thioridazine and glutethimide were prescribed in quantities sufficient for two weeks. Three days later the patient returned and requested more medication from the internist. When this was refused, the patient became extremely agitated. He was eventually given a two-week supply of ethchorvynol for sleep. Three days later the patient returned and requested paraldehyde, but this was refused. Six days later he insistently demanded more medication and was given meprobamate and chloral hydrate, on condition that he accept referrals to the psychiatric clinic at the local hospital. He visited the psychiatric outpatient department on several occasions and received a variety of psychopharmaceuticals from that unit as well.
>
> The patient continued his near-violent approach to obtaining tranquilizers and hypnotics. Finally it was necessary to tell him that the shelter clinic staff was no longer allowed to write such prescriptions.
>
> Subsequently the patient began to complain of pruritis. He succeeded in eliciting a prescription for diphenhydramine hydrochloride. When renewals of medication were refused, the patient began to complain of a cough, for which he received elixir of terpin hydrate with codeine.
>
> This patient succeeded in manipulating clinic personnel despite major efforts to counsel him and to place him in a more appropriate program for treatment of his emotional disorder, alcoholism, and drug dependence.[30]

Awareness of this phenomenon has helped teams to locate and care for these types of patients effectively.[10,15,17]

Questions of confidentiality are potential problems for patients as well as team members. This is controlled by a clear commitment among team members and an understanding by the patient that the team functions as an entity. All information is shared so that confidentiality is preserved within the team's boundaries rather than by individual members.[15,17] Finally, potential patient problems provoked by the use of a team approach may be addressed through patient education and a heightened team awareness of such issues.

The experience of learning from and giving to professional colleagues is one that calls upon all of one's resources as a professional and as a human being. It necessitates for all a high level of commitment and involvement. Many are the moments of frustration and misunderstanding. But when it all comes together and the team works smoothly and efficiently, it can be exhilarating. It is at these times that interdisciplinary team work offers patients the very best in primary comprehensive medical care.[17]

REFERENCES

1. Brickner, PW. Home health care for the aged. New York: Appleton-Century-Crofts, 1978.
2. Dienst ER, Byl N. Evaluation of an educational program in health care teams. J Comm Health. 1981; 6:4.
3. Barber JH, Kratz CR. Towards team care. New York: Churchill Livingstone, 1980.
4. Gibson RW. Mental health and primary medical care. Group for the Advancement of Psychiatry, Publication 10:699, 1980.
5. Knopke HJ, Diekelmann NL. Approaches to teaching primary health care. St. Louis: CV Mosby Co., 1981.
6. Elliot A. The primary health care team. Nursing Focus. 1980; 2:3.
7. Wise H, Beckhard R, Rubin I, Kyte A. Making health teams work. Cambridge, Mass.: Ballinger, 1974.
8. Doron H. Developing concepts and patterns of primary care. Israel J Med Sciences. 1983; 19:81.
9. Eshelman FN, Campagna K. Pharmaceutical services for the primary health care team. Hosp Pharmacy. 1976; 11:8.
10. Ducanis AJ, Golin AK. The interdisciplinary health care team. Germantown, Md.: Aspen Systems, 1979.
11. Thompson TL, Byzny R. Primary and team health care education. New York: Praeger, 1983.
12. Shukla RB: The role of primary care team in the care of the elderly. The Practitioner. 1981; 225:1356.
13. Brooks D, Hendy A, Parsonage A. Towards the reality of the primary health care team: an educational approach. J Royal Coll Gen Practitioners. 1981; 31:229.
14. Saint-Yves IF. Teamwork within the primary health team. Royal Soc Health J. 1982; 102:232.
15. Savarese M. Interdisciplinary teams. Transcript from workshop on Health Issues in Care for the Homeless Conference, New York, October 1983.
16. Beales G. Making the team work. Nursing Mirror. 1981; 153:11.
17. Lee S. Interdisciplinary teaming in primary care: a process of evolution and resolution. Social Work in Health Care. 1980; 5:3.

18. Rubin IM, Plovinick MS, Fry RE. Improving the coordination of care: a program for health team development. Cambridge, Mass.: Ballinger, 1975.
19. Gross AM, Gross H, Eisenstein-Naveh RA. Defining the role of the social worker in primary health care. Health and Social Work. 1983; 8:3.
20. Milne MA. The primary health team: linked group discussion as a learning medium. J Advanced Nursing. 1981; 6:5.
21. LaMontagne DR. Teamwork makes a difference in urban health center. Commitment. 1977; 3:7.
22. Bowling A. Teamwork in primary health care. Nursing Times. 1983; 79:48.
23. Rabkin MT. Patient-centered teamwork is focus of new primary care program. Hosp Med Staff. 1977; 6:6.
24. Hart LL, Evans DC, Welker RG, Frits JN: The clinical pharmacist on an interdisciplinary primary health care team. Drug Intelligence and Clinical Pharmacy. 1979; 13:7–8.
25. Bachrach LL. Continuity of care for chronic mental patients: a conceptual analysis. Am J Psych. 1981; 138:11.
26. Schwartz SR, Goldman HH, Shoshanna C. Case management for the chronic mentally ill: models and dimensions. Hosp & Comm Psych. 1982; 33:12.
27. Fawcett-Henesy AR. Teamwork that pays dividends. Nursing Mirror. 1981; 153:25.
28. Cunningham RM. Making the patient a partner. Am Med News. 1978; 21:12.
29. Greene JY, Weinberger M, Mamlin JJ. Patient attitudes toward health care: expectations of primary care in a clinical setting. Soc Sci Med. 1980; Part A, 14:2.
30. Brickner PW, Greenbaum D, Kaufman A, et al. A clinic for male derelicts. Ann Int Med. 1972; 77:565–69.

18

Working with Hospitals

Linda Keen Scharer and Bart Price

When homeless people require treatment at hospitals for acute or chronic conditions, problems relating to admission, compliance, length of stay, and payment for service often follow. Successful resolution of these matters varies with the individual patient's condition, the hospital chosen, and communication among all those involved in the care required. A review of the hospital's function and discussions with administrators and workers at shelter sites, hospitals, and government offices reveal the dimensions of the issues and provide specific suggestions for improving care of the homeless.

At the center of the practice of modern medicine is the hospital. Although hospitals have been praised as sites where the latest in medical advances and patient care are available, they have also been attacked for the arrogance of their physicians, the dehumanization of their patients, and, most of all, the cost of their services.

In an effort to control costs, government payers for service use various cost-containment procedures, such as reducing the number of beds, limiting the length of a patient's stay, and instituting and enforcing stringent reimbursement policies. Particularly affected by such measures are urban hospitals, the traditional focus of care for the poor and the homeless. Unacceptable staff behavior and limitations on hospital resources affect all those who enter hospitals, but the homeless are particularly vulnerable because they strain the system through their behavior, medical indigency, and anticipated length of stay.

In an effort to understand and thereby reduce the real barriers in treating the homeless, two workshops were convened at the conference on Health Issues for the Homeless, sponsored by St. Vincent's Hospital and the United Hospital Fund of New York. In general, participants (see Appendix) represented three groups: caregivers employed at shelters, hospital administrators, and hospital-based outreach staff.

Information shared during these workshops stimulated further research and additional interviews. The results are reported here under the following points:

- Descriptions of the homeless patient;
- Expectations for hospital care;
- Perspectives of hospital employees;
- Strategies for successful hospital use;
- Possible alternatives to hospital use;
- Limitations in providing health care at hospitals.

DESCRIPTIONS OF THE HOMELESS PATIENT

A homeless patient cannot be stereotyped. Patients using a hospital clinic may include a 13-year-old delinquent who has been banished from home to live on the streets, a 32-year-old man who requires drug detoxification, or a 77-year-old woman who is suffering from the ills of old age as well as exposure.

The perception remains that, as a group, the homeless are physically unattractive and perhaps considered unworthy of care because of their unusual and sometimes bizarre behavior. Consider the following comments from workshop participants:

> I think the patients are disliked as a population. I think they are being punished by a total society not merely an institution.

> He's had a chance at life and messed it up. You and your friend get the hell out of here because I'm responsible for taking in the people who have heart attacks.

> I myself have felt when I've seen men drinking Thunderbird in front of me . . . I have thought, my tax dollars for their Thunderbird.

> I think a lot of the people treating those people have alcoholism problems themselves or their fathers and mothers have been alcoholics.

Each hospital and each shelter site should know the general demographic characteristics of the people they serve, as well as the type of medical services they require. Awareness of age, sex, race, cultural differences, and environment permits intelligent planning for staff recruitment and implementation of medical services.

EXPECTATIONS FOR HOSPITAL CARE

Public image and need make the hospital appear to be a logical shelter for the homeless even when acute medical conditions do not exist. In part, this perception results from the absence of other effective resources.[1] In addition, the past behavior of those who founded and administered hospitals is consistent with a promise of help. Hospitals have been looked upon as the alternative to family care, and homeless individuals become part of this family.[2]

Thus the concept of the hospital as a shelter comes from examples in recent history, the religious sponsorship of particular institutions, and the failure of others to provide care.

The almshouses of the nineteenth century provided a haven and gave medical care if needed. Hospitals are extensions of the almshouses, a phenomenon not confined to public hospitals but extended into the practices of voluntary institutions.[3] Unwed mothers, for example, could find refuge and food as well as medical care at selected New York City hospitals in the late nineteenth and early twentieth centuries.[4]

Hospitals sponsored by religious orders bring with them the tradition of caring for both body and spirit, and these hospitals are the manifestation of biblical edicts.[5] In particular, religious orders have demonstrated interest in promoting hospitals for the sick poor. Members of the order then are able to carry out the work of Christ and provide a source of employment for themselves.[6]

In the days of philanthropic and religious support, hospital care could be devoted to the poor. Now, at the end of the twentieth century, people enter hospitals for treatment of defined problems for specific periods of time. They are expected to pay for their care through either insurance or their own resources.

PERSPECTIVES OF HOSPITAL EMPLOYEES

Those working with the homeless have different impressions of the problem, depending on their function in the organization of care.

Hospitals are composed of many types and levels of personnel. There are those with whom the patient has direct contact, such as doctors, nurses, aides, and social workers; and there are those, such as the administrative staff, whose work shapes patient care activities but who do not necessarily have direct contact with patients. In order for the patient to have a successful stay, admitting clerks, nurses, house staff, aides, utilization review committees, and business office administrators have to maintain a harmonious approach.

The strongest case for hospitalization of the homeless occurs when the need is clear-cut: the organization has a prior commitment to the homeless, financial arrangements are possible, the patient is compliant, the case is medically interesting, and there is a place for the patient to return upon discharge. Otherwise, one encounters a number of possible scenarios. There is the case of the disgruntled house officer who is not learning about diseases, the nurse caring for unappreciative patients, trustees worrying about the reputation of the hospital; most troublesome, there are the concerns of the financial officers.

Even when financial eligibility is established, length of stay becomes a significant problem. Hospitals, while charitable enterprises, must adjust to state and federal payment systems if they are to survive. Extended stays can occur because of difficulties in discharge planning. One hospital's Director of Quality Assurance put it this way:

> All the people involved in homeless programs have stressed the amount of time that it takes to secure the confidence of homeless people so that they will be allowed to try to help them. This is the one commodity that the hospitalized patient does not have. There is not the kind of time to allow the people responsible for discharge planning to get the acceptance of the patients to help them.

In the end, the financial perspective may be the controlling factor.

Yet, it is important to recognize that all employees can have an impact on the care the homeless receive. In at least one institution, hands-on-care personnel have advocated and perhaps changed the institutional attitude, as a remark made by a hospital financial officer indicates:

> If you hang around long enough with these people from Community Medicine, they'll break you down.

STRATEGIES FOR SUCCESSFUL HOSPITAL USE

Perhaps the best way to demonstrate how hospitals can be utilized successfully by homeless patients is to cite an example. The following experiences were related at the conference by a social worker at Yale–New Haven Hospital.

> New Haven has two hospitals; one of them, my institution, has traditionally served the indigent, the homeless, the poor, any classification of uncovered patient.
>
> Over a period of years the emergency room seemed to be the place, as in most institutions, where we found homeless patients. The police brought them in beginning about five years ago, after alcoholism was decriminalized. It turned out to be a Police Department to emergency room problem. We worked collaboratively in New Haven: ambulance companies, community agencies, and the hospital, predominantly the social work department, and all of us worked with the city welfare department obtaining grant money to create a shelter.
>
> It took about two years to bring about the shelter but it was achieved through the efforts of a great many organizations within New Haven. Once we brought it about we stayed together on it. This was an invaluable lesson for me. The working relationships had to stay together for the success of the shelter. New people came in, the ambulance companies and the police backed out, and we started to prospect, i.e., to find new, now appropriate, sources of assistance. We asked community action agencies to help us find housing; we asked the city social work department to help the shelter folk do discharge planning. We made friends with people in temporary labor, the rehabilitation department, and employment office. These collaborative relationships give the caregivers some sense of mutual interest, a sense of support and acknowledgement.
>
> Throughout the hospital, I am now identified as the contact

person and it is invaluable. For example, the secretary for one of our administrators saw a homeless couple sitting in a park right near the shelter, and she wanted to know what was going on. I was called and I knew what they were doing there. The woman was visiting her mother who was in the hospital, and her husband—like any good son-in-law who didn't like his mother-in-law—was waiting downstairs with a shopping cart and two large suitcases. It's not unusual for me to be called. We have a security department. They are really top drawer. They know that I'm the person who is the contact for people who don't look like they really belong to any particular network.

We talk about sensitizing caregivers. We let the doctors, nurses, and social workers know what home situation the person in the shelter has. Then there are all the ancillary people: the clerk who checks them in, the clinic admitting clerk, the secretary to the administrator.

All of these are important issues and one person should be identified and constantly working on them. You don't deal with the homeless twice a year or every three months: you are identified in the hospital newsletter and a variety of other ways as the person folks should contact.

This experience shows that there are at least five steps necessary to plan for effective hospital use.

1. Make the hospital a part of early planning for the homeless.
2. Identify one person at an institution to address all questions about the homeless.
3. When working with others at a hospital, be aware of their concerns.
4. Maintain communication with all relevant members of the hospital community.
5. Have modest expectations for achievement.

While each step presents its own degree of difficulty, the fourth can be particularly elusive. For example, one of the outreach workers at a hospital with a well-developed program noted that there were three key people from her own hospital that she had never met. She concluded:

We have to aggressively seek each other out and know who we are and know that we're all on the same side and attempt to work something pragmatically together.

POSSIBLE ALTERNATIVES TO
HOSPITAL USE

There is a general trend to use less hospitalization for the care and diagnosis of disease, and services for homeless patients are being affected by this trend. One sees an example of this general trend in the establishment of outpatient, short-stay surgery units. The hospital is still used, but a less intensive form of hospital care is selected. Similar practices exist now under special conditions. A pediatrician explained:

> We're able to keep them from hospitalization days because we are sure that person is going to come back to us in three days and we can take care of them on an outpatient basis.

Hospital use for the homeless is reduced when alternative places for care and shelter are found. Implicit in the approach is giving as much care as possible outside the institution, either at satellite clinics or at a shelter itself. The Mercy Hospice, working with the Hall–Mercer Mental Health Center in Philadelphia, is one example of this practice, the benefits of which are described below:

> Most of the women at the shelter have always tended to be afraid of psychiatry or of getting any kind of intervention. I think by being in the shelter and by my presence out on the street, in my blue jeans, my giving them food and other kinds of services as a warm-up has allowed them to begin to trust a little bit and come into the shelter, and eventually get the type of mental health care that they needed.

The next view on patient care comes from the shelter administrator:

> It gives us the chance to work with the mothers, as mothers with children, because Hall–Mercer is able to send their workers right into our shelters; because they are there steadily, we find we are able to serve them a lot more effectively.

In addition, satellite clinics or hospitals can offer twenty-four-hour access to an emergency room hotline and in-service training for shelter staff. It is the cycle of discharge to the streets without appropriate medical follow-up that leads to readmission for treatment of a previously seen medical condition. At other times the answer may be admission to a nursing home or a state mental hospital. Specially targeted funds for health care—acute, chronic, long-term—were recommended as the steps to encourage alternative care before and after discharge. Consider the following comment:

> Most of the people who have been hospitalized in our acute care unit from the street sleep most of the time, sleep and eat, and don't use the multimillion dollar facility.

Alternatives to hospital use can be stimulated by shifting the focus of fund raising. An administrator from a New Orleans hospital describes the process:

> We went for funding of the network itself, not leaving out any of the agencies—police department, coroner's office, Charity Hospital travelers' aid—and we got funding for the network.

Therefore, no one agency such as the hospital has a turf imperative. This wider constituency has political implications.

> Through the effort of the network we've been able to pull in our politicians within the area because we have a city, state, nonprofit link.

A final prerequisite to encouraging care is easy access to Medicaid. In 1980 and 1981 agencies in many states could easily obtain Medicaid for homeless individuals. This practice has become more restricted. However, with this source of funds, social services and other forms of medical care outside hospitals would readily be available, because the recipient would not be a charity case.

Sometimes the alternative of no hospital use is the last resort. In the words of one shelter worker:

> A lot of time I just have to abandon the effort. You almost have to say the street is better or suggest the Number 7 train is much better.

LIMITATIONS IN PROVIDING CARE AT HOSPITALS

The major limitations in providing hospital care are the wishes of the patient, the number of hospitals available to give such care,[7] and financial reimbursement practices.[8] Once inside, the homeless may leave before care is completed:

> You don't have to be very bright to know that the homeless are
> difficult to place. Why should you bother to admit them in the first
> place?

It is a preconception that in urban settings one hospital is responsible for the care of the indigent. However, information received from forty-two of the most populous cities in the United States shows that 55 percent indicated the presence of more than one hospital willing to take care of the homeless.[9] Twenty-one percent of the hospitals were public and 71 percent were voluntary.[10] It is possible that changes for the worse may be taking place: since the number of public hospitals closing in recent years is well documented, some cities may be left without adequate acute care institutions to care for the homeless. Certainly in cities with only one hospital accepting responsibility there are fewer avenues of care for those people.

Reimbursement by diagnostic related groups (DRGs) directs hospitals to discharge patients within the prescribed time for their individual diagnosis, because when a patient's stay exceeds the limit set, there is effectively no more reimbursement to the hospital. If the hospital then insists that the homeless patient leave, the consequences are harsh.

Under this system, however, if a hospital can cut costs, it is allowed to keep the money saved. DRGs make possible a redistribution of dollars; therefore in theory the money saved could be used to subsidize charity care.[11]

This phenomenon would permit hospitals with a history of mission for the poor and/or those who felt the pressure of political realities to give care without financial hardship. The situation described below would be avoided:

> A couple of years ago we kept a homeless patient in the hospital
> and attempted to make a community plan. We had days denied
> for reimbursement and when we went to argue we were told very
> directly: you are not the caretakers of humanity. You may choose
> to be but we can choose not to pay you to do it.

With adequate financial reimbursement, responsive to inflation, humane discharge planning is possible. One must be cautious, however, because government funding agencies in the past have been quick to reduce discretionary funds. Caretakers and other interested parties take heed.

While modest gains are possible, further expectation for acceptance of the homeless person for hospital care depends upon modification of federal policies of reimbursement and changes in treatment practices.

APPENDIX

Gay Lynn Bond, Director of Social Services, Charity Hospital, New Orleans

Susan Caldwell, Staff Therapist, Outpatient Department, Hall–Mercer Mental Health and Mental Retardation Center, Philadelphia

Sylvia Grey, Director of Patient Accounts, St. Vincent's Hospital and Medical Center of New York

Mary Ann Lee, Pediatrician, Primary Care Program, St. Vincent's Hospital and Medical Center of New York

Mary Jean O'Brien, Nursing Supervisor, Department of Community Medicine, St. Vincent's Hospital and Medical Center of New York

Frank O'Connor, Social Worker, Primary Care Center, Yale–New Haven Hospitals

Barbara Olvany, Director of Quality Assurance, St. Vincent's Hospital and Medical Center of New York

Sr. Kathleen Schneider, Administrator, Mercy Hospital, Philadelphia

Angel Vergez, Assistant Director of Patient Accounts, St. Vincent's Hospital and Medical Center of New York

The sessions were moderated by:

Bart Price, Vice President, Finance, Yale–New Haven Hospitals

Linda Keen Scharer, Assistant Director, Department of Community Medicine, St. Vincent's Hospital and Medical Center of New York

REFERENCES

1. Rodgers D, Blenden RJ. The academic medical center: a stressed American institution. N Engl J Med. 1978; 298:940–50.
2. Starr P. The transformation of American medicine. New York: Basic Books, 1982; 145–79.
3. Ibid: 149.
4. Rosner D. A once charitable enterprise—hospitals and health care in Brooklyn and New York, 1885–1915. New York: Cambridge University Press, 1982:4.
5. Matthew 8:1–18, Mark 1:29.
6. Glaser W. Social setting and medical organization: a cross national study of the hospital. New York: Atherton Press, 1970.
7. Issacs MR, Lichter K, Lipshulz C. The urban public hospital options for the 1980s. Bethesda, Md.: Alpha Center, August 1982.
8. Hadley J, Mullner R, Feder J. The financially distressed hospital. N Engl J Med. 1982; 307:1283–87.

9. Unpublished information from cities.
10. American hospital association guide to the health care field, 1983 edition. Chicago, Ill.
11. Igelhart JK. New era of prospective reimbursement for hospitals. N Engl J Med. 1982; 307:1289.

19

A Public Hospital in a Community Network of Services for the Homeless: The Role of Charity Hospital, New Orleans

Gay Lynn Bond, Karen Wilkinson, and Monica Mang

A public hospital has an important role in health care for the homeless and, through its Social Service Department, can serve as a major link in a community network of services for these people. Charity Hospital at New Orleans (CHNO) is part of such a network. This network, and Charity Hospital's role within it, is influenced by the unique characteristics of the city. These include the cultural and social structure and the system of social services currently in existence.

THE CITY AND ITS PRIMARY SERVICE PROVIDERS

New Orleans, Louisiana, is the twenty-first largest city in the United States, nestled within a bend near the mouth of the Mississippi River. The weather is humid and rainy, particularly during the summer and early fall months; the seasonal temperatures are moderate.

The 1980 census reports the population of the New Orleans metropolitan area to be 1,078,588.[1] There are more females (53.25 percent) than males, and a greater percentage of blacks (56.42 percent) than whites.[1] The median annual income in 1979 was $15,615 for individuals and $18,033 for families. The per capita income, however, was $7,141.[1] An estimated 4000 homeless people live in New Orleans.[2] A large number of this group have come from elsewhere seeking employment. The Sunbelt is perceived to be an area of great job opportunities. Although New Orleans may be growing, the city has suffered economically along with the rest of the nation in the recent recession. As a result, state funds for social programs have been cut, reducing the number of employees and efforts to help the poor and homeless.

Several charitable organizations offer services that attempt to meet these needs. There are five shelters that provide a total of 580 beds each night.[3,4] They are: the Baptist Rescue Mission (187 beds—20 for women); the Ozanam Inn, operated by the Brothers of the Good Shepherd (86 beds); the Salvation Army Men's Lodge and Women's Lodge (115 and 22 beds, respectively); and the Care Center, which opened in March 1984 and provides 20 beds for women and children. The shelters are located in the skid row area, except those for women only. The four shelters that were open in 1983 provided shelter 157,663 times.[5] These shelters are full to capacity 95 to 100 percent of the time; they are often over capacity during the winter.[5] Lines for beds begin to form in the late afternoon. By 7:00 P.M. most of the shelters are full and must turn people away.[5] Homeless people must then search for a safe place to sleep and often end up roaming the streets all night. In New Orleans, it is against the law for a person to sleep in a park, in a vehicle, on a sidewalk, or on city-owned property. The New Orleans police arrested 646 people for ''sleeping on public property'' in 1983.[5] The penalty is a fine up to $100 or a jail sentence of up to ninety days.

Single-room-occupancy (SRO) hotels offer low rental rates for those who can afford them. An estimated 320 to 420 rooms are available in the skid row area. These hotels are often frequented by the transients who work on the docks and ships in the port of New Orleans.[6] The downtown YMCA also offers low-rent rooms, but most are rented by visiting international students.

The Baptist Rescue Mission, the Ozanam Inn, both Salvation Army lodges, and the Felicity United Methodist Church (on Sunday evening only) serve meals to the homeless. The Emergency Assistance of Associated Catholic Charities also provides food supplies for transients.[7] Approximately 470,000 meals were served by these agencies in 1983.[8]

Several of these programs provide clothing to the homeless.[9] The

Social Service Department at Charity Hospital also provides free clothing to those patients in need.

The Salvation Army offers counseling, job training, job placement, and transportation to job sites. Through this program 3070 persons found jobs in 1983. Domestic counseling, an Alcoholics Anonymous program, and a follow-up program on all persons counseled are also offered by this agency.[10] The Travelers Aid Society helps newcomers to New Orleans, including homeless individuals who come looking for work. The agency has a counseling and job placement service and has secured permanent employment for over 400 people within the last year. Travelers Aid also supplies up to nine days of shelter and food for the homeless. From June 1983 to March 1984, 4531 shelter nights and 5236 meals were provided.[11]

The Baptist Mission, Ozanam Inn, Travelers Aid Society, and Salvation Army are resources for temporary relief. While these agencies offer counseling and placement programs, their major goal is to provide the basics—food, shelter, and clothing. The agencies are not equipped to manage the needs of all the clients they serve. The current system of services lacks a central referral and follow-up body that can identify the long range needs of each person and work with that person to satisfy those needs.

L'HÔPITAL DES PAUVRES DE LA CHARITE

What role should a public hospital play in the network of community resources that provide aid to the homeless? Let us look at CHNO's contribution to the system of services offered in New Orleans.

Charity is the oldest and largest of the nine state-owned and operated hospitals in Louisiana. The primary mission of these institutions is to give health care to the indigent population throughout the state.

Today, Charity has approximately 6000 employees[14] and 1500 licensed beds, averages 35,000 admissions per year, and treats an average of 18,220 patients per month through the emergency room and outpatient clinics.[15] (See Table 19.1.) The emergency rooms and walk-in clinic are the primary access areas for the homeless population in New Orleans.

Charity Hospital offers the widest range of services and provides most of the health care to the homeless population of New Orleans. It is within walking distance of skid row. The shelters usually refer their

Table 19.1.   Charity Hospital at New Orleans Statistics, Fiscal Year 1982–83 and Fiscal Year 1983–84 (New Orleans, Louisiana March, 1984)

	FY 1982–83	FY 1983–84 (July 1983–February 1984)
Licensed beds	1,500	1,500
Staffed beds	1,085	1,050
Occupancy rate	76.4%	77.7%
Number of admissions	35,194	23,176
Inpatient days	303,270	199,370
Average length of stay	8.6 days	8.3 days
Number of Emergency Room Cases	176,611	133,233
Number of Outpatient Clinic visits	443,136	297,300

residents in need of medical attention to Charity. The New Orleans police transport most persons they find on the street who appear to need medical, psychiatric, or detoxification services to Charity Hospital. See Table 19.2 for sources of referral.

The Wetmore Clinic, Veterans Administration Hospital, and the mental health centers serve as other sources of health care for the homeless of New Orleans. Wetmore Clinic performed 3280 chest x-rays on homeless individuals in 1983 and is currently treating fifty-two homeless tuberculous patients.[12] Most of the shelters require persons applying for beds to have a tuberculosis screening test.

Of the 5670 persons being treated in the area mental health centers, an estimated 1500 are homeless. Not included are those patients in the Charity Hospital psychiatric units, private institutions, or state institutions serving the catchment area.[13]

THE HOMELESS POPULATION SERVED AT CHNO

A study aimed at identifying the composition of the homeless, the number of patient visits made, and the types of services provided to these patients was recently perfoi.ned at Charity Hospital.

A total of 20,011 patient route sheets from the emergency room and walk-in clinic for the months of January and February 1984 were reviewed. The route sheets were obtained from the patient accounts division of the Department of Finance and represented those accounts that had been entered into the computer billing system. Each record was judged against a set of criteria, and 432 were determined to represent visits by homeless individuals. Patient data was extracted from those route sheets, the information was tabulated, and the results are represented in Tables 19.3–19.9.

There were several deficiencies within the data collection system used:

1. Because data collectors had access only to those route sheets that had been entered into the billing system, not all patient records were available.

2. Many patients left without treatment, taking their route sheets with them. The record of their request for medical help was lost.[16–18]

3. A complete list of SRO hotels in the New Orleans area was not available. Therefore, not all homeless who gave an SRO address were identified.

4. Those patients without an address might not have been homeless and other information—age, sex, race, major complaint—might not have been accurate.

5. The physician's diagnosis was not always available and might have differed from the patient's major complaint.

6. Many patients gave false addresses. The addresses of sixty pa-

Table 19.2. Sources of Referral—Addresses Stated on Homeless Patient Records, January and February, 1984 (Emergency Room and Walk-in Clinic Visits, Charity Hospital at New Orleans, Louisiana, 1984)

	Number	Percentage
General delivery	51	11.81
Baptist Mission	83	19.21
Ozanam Inn	43	9.95
Salvation Army	16	3.70
YMCA	9	2.08
Out of town	36	8.33
No address given	84	19.44
Two addresses given	41	9.49
Other	69	15.97
Total:	432	99.98

Table 19.3.   Number and Percentage of Homeless Patient
Records Reviewed, Race by Sex, January and February,
1984 (Charity Hospital at New Orleans, Louisiana, 1984)

	Male	Female	Total
Black	115 (26.6%)	77 (17.8%)	192 (44.4%)
Other	11 (2.5%)	2 (.5%)	13 (3.0%)
White	197 (45.6%)	30 (6.9%)	227 (52.5%)
Total:	323 (74.7%)	109 (25.2%)	432 (99.9%)

tients treated on a particular day were looked up in the city's telephone-
address cross-reference directory. Forty of the sixty were bogus. While
it cannot be assumed that only homeless people gave false addresses,
those homeless patients who did give a false address were unidentified
and therefore excluded from the survey.

7. Any homeless patients taken directly to the Crisis Intervention
Unit (CIU) were also excluded from the survey.

FROM THE HOSPITAL
TO THE COMMUNITY

The Social Work Services (SWS) Department links the hospital with
the community's network of available social service resources. The mission of its program is the development and maintenance of a flexible
program of services directed toward strengthening patients' coping
skills and maximizing their ability to function independently. The main
elements of the program include:

- Development of a continuum of social services ranging from preventive to follow-up intervention;
- Participation as professional members of the interdisciplinary patient care team and provision of educational input regarding Social Service's role at Charity and pertinent aspects of social work
  practice;
- Assessment, coordination, and development of necessary community systems and resources that affect the delivery of services
  to patients of Charity Hospital;
- Evaluation of social services through the continued development
  of an internal quality assurance program.

Table 19.4. Percentages of Male Homeless Patient Visits through CHNO Emergency Room and Walk-in Clinic, Race by Age, January and February, 1984 (Charity Hospital at New Orleans, Louisiana, 1984)

Total		0–25	26–35	36–45	46–55	56–65	66–75	75+	No Information
100%	Black	13.04%	21.74%	33.91%	16.52%	6.09%	3.48%	2.61%	2.61%
99.99%	Other	27.27%	27.27%	18.18%	9.09%	0	0	0	18.18%
99.99%	White	10.15%	37.56%	18.78%	16.75%	12.69%	1.52%	0	2.54%

Table 19.5. Percentages of Female Homeless Patient Visits through CHNO Emergency Room and Walk-in Clinic, Race by Age, January and February, 1984 (Charity Hospital at New Orleans, Louisiana, 1984)

	0–25	26–35	36–45	46–55	56–65	66–75	75+	No Information	Total
Black	36.36%	37.66%	10.39%	2.60%	3.90%	2.60%	5.19%	1.30%	100%
Other	50.00%	0	50.00%	0	0	0	0	0	100%
White	46.67%	20.00%	6.67%	6.67%	6.67%	0	6.66%	6.66%	100%

At Charity Hospital, the Social Work Services program has the primary responsibility of tapping community resources to meet the needs of the patients referred to the department, and it strives to meet that responsibility as part of an open referral system. Physicians made slightly less than one-half of the referrals in fiscal year 1982–83. Nurse referrals and patient self-referrals composed over a third of the total patients seen, and the rest were referred by other sources, including community agencies. The open referral system has its problems: the referring source may not be aware of the patient's homeless status, perceive a social problem the patient has that could affect his discharge, or know about the Social Work Services program at Charity Hospital. The result is that not all homeless persons treated at CHNO are reached by SWS; its coverage at nights and on weekends is limited. Charity's open door policy and tradition of refusing treatment to no one creates a demand for the medical services that at times is difficult to meet. Most care and treatment must be provided through emergency areas and outpatient clinics. The criteria for admission are strict and often exceed those of private hospitals in the community: one's medical condition must require ongoing attention by physicians and nurses. Homeless individuals frequently have noncritical conditions and are seldom admitted. Those who are not admitted still have health problems and other needs that must be addressed.

SWS has some specific programs and services to aid the homeless. Trust funds, community monies, and donations are used to provide indigent patients with necessary medication, appliances, and transportation. Volunteer Services provides free clothing to those in need. SWS can obtain free sandwiches and milk through the dietary department for people who are hungry. As part of one formal program, it purchases and distributes twenty-five tickets for beds each month at the Baptist Mission shelter. The cost is $3.75 per night.

Another internal program is the Emergency Medical Services (EMS) automatic referral for repeaters. In 1976, the EMS-Outpatient Unit staff began to identify a group of patients who made repeated visits to the emergency room primarily for social rather than medical problems. Social workers met with emergency room nursing and physician staff, compiled a list of current EMS repeaters, and devised criteria to identify future EMS repeaters. A system to divert these patients to the EMS-Outpatient Unit was developed.

Approximately one-third of the EMS repeaters rely on the EMS-Outpatient Unit for social support and move in and out of homelessness. These cases are generally complex in nature. A treatment plan is developed. The unit worker assigned accepts the responsibility for ongoing case management of that EMS repeater. When a placement

Table 19.6. Percentages of Homeless Black Male Patient Visits through CHNO Emergency Room and Walk-in Clinic, Age by Major Complaint, January and February, 1984 (Charity Hospital at New Orleans, Louisiana)

					Major Complaint				
Age	(# of visits)	Back (%)	Chest/ Heart (%)	Eye (%)	Frost- bite (%)	Gastric (%)	Gyn (%)	Leg & Feet (%)	Mental (%)
0–25	(14)	—	—	—	—	7.14	—	14.29	14.29
26–35	(25)	—	—	—	—	8.00	—	—	24.00
36–45	(37)	—	5.41	2.70	2.70	8.11	—	8.11	2.70
46–55	(18)	5.55	16.67	—	—	5.55	—	5.56	5.56
56–65	(8)	—	—	—	—	—	—	25.00	—
66–75	(3)	—	—	—	—	—	—	—	—
76+	(2)	—	50.0	—	—	—	—	50.00	—
Not available	(2)	—	—	—	—	—	—	—	—

breaks down, clients often return to the EMS-Outpatient Unit for case management coordination of another plan.

Since homeless individuals typically require an array of services that the hospital alone cannot provide, Charity Social Work Services works to increase its awareness of community resources and maintains a close working relationship with the thirty-nine social agencies that assist the homeless. A formal management program has been designed

Table 19.7. Percentages of Homeless White Male Patient Visits through CHNO Emergency Room and Walk-in Clinic, Age by Major Complaint, January and February, 1984 (Charity Hospital at New Orleans, Louisiana)

					Major Complaint				
Age	(# of visits)	Back (%)	Chest/ Heart (%)	Eye (%)	Frost- bite (%)	Gastric (%)	Gyn (%)	Leg & Feet (%)	Mental (%)
0–25	(21)	—	4.76	4.76	—	4.76	—	14.29	4.76
26–35	(74)	—	6.76	4.05	1.35	8.11	—	9.46	18.92
36–45	(36)	—	—	5.56	2.78	2.78	—	11.11	8.33
46–55	(33)	—	12.12	3.03	—	3.03	—	6.06	—
56–65	(25)	—	4.00	—	—	16.00	—	—	20.00
66–75	(3)	—	—	—	—	—	—	33.33	—
76+	(0)	—	—	—	—	—	—	—	—
Not available	(4)	—	25.00	—	—	—	—	25.00	—

Table 19.6. Continued

| | Major Complaint | | | | | | | |
OB (%)	Respira-tory (%)	Seizures (%)	Skin (%)	Substance Abuse (%)	Teeth (%)	Trauma (%)	Other (%)	Total (%)
—	7.14	—	—	14.29	—	21.43	21.42	100.00
—	8.00	—	—	4.00	—	20.00	36.00	100.00
—	21.62	18.92	—	8.11	—	10.81	10.81	100.00
—	5.55	5.56	—	11.11	—	22.22	16.67	100.00
—	—	13.00	12.00	13.00	—	12.00	25.00	100.00
—	—	—	—	100.00	—	—	—	100.00
—	—	—	—	—	—	—	—	100.00
—	50.00	—	—	—	—	50.00	—	100.00

to systematize SWS's relationship with these agencies. CHNO's internal committee system aids in the assessment, coordination, and development of necessary community systems and resources that affect the delivery of services to the patients at Charity. Staff members who sit on the committees are assigned a related cluster of community service agencies and act as liaison. For example, members of the Patient Placement Committee must be aware of developments, new agencies, and changing admission requirements of nursing homes, shelters, boarding homes, group homes, and state institutions. The committee members

Table 19.7. Continued

| | Major Complaint | | | | | | | |
OB (%)	Respira-tory (%)	Seizures (%)	Skin (%)	Substance Abuse (%)	Teeth (%)	Trauma (%)	Other (%)	Total (%)
—	4.76	—	9.52	4.76	—	23.81	23.81	99.99
—	9.46	1.35	1.35	8.11	2.70	13.51	14.86	99.99
—	2.78	2.78	11.11	22.22	2.78	19.44	8.33	100.00
—	9.09	9.09	—	21.21	—	15.15	21.21	99.99
—	4.00	4.00	—	8.00	—	20.00	24.00	100.00
—	—	—	—	33.33	—	33.33	—	99.99
—	—	—	—	—	—	—	—	—
—	—	—	—	—	—	50.00	—	100.00

Table 19.8.   Percentages of Homeless Black Female Patient Visits through CHNO Emergency Room and Walk-in Clinic, Age by Major Complaint, January and February, 1984 (Charity Hospital at New Orleans, Louisiana)

Age	(#of visits)	Back (%)	Chest/ Heart (%)	Eye (%)	Frost- bite (%)	Gastric (%)	Gyn (%)	Leg & Feet (%)	Mental (%)
0–25	(28)	—	—	—	—	17.86	14.29	14.29	3.59
26–35	(28)	—	17.86	7.14	—	3.57	17.86	—	14.29
36–45	(8)	25.00	—	12.00	—	—	—	—	—
46–55	(3)	—	—	—	—	33.33	—	33.33	—
56–65	(3)	—	66.66	—	—	—	—	—	—
66–75	(2)	50.00	—	—	—	50.00	—	—	—
76+	(4)	—	75.00	—	—	—	—	—	25.00
Not available	(1)	100.00	—	—	—	—	—	—	—

receive calls from and meet with agency representatives and disseminate relevant information concerning the agencies to the rest of the staff.

Social Work Services has tried through its committee structure to develop community resources for placement for the homeless and other patients with inadequate living/housing arrangements. This ex-

Table 19.9.   Percentages of Homeless White Female Patient Visits through CHNO Emergency Room and Walk-in Clinic, Age by Major Complaint, January and February, 1984 (Charity Hospital at New Orleans, Louisiana)

Age	(# of visits)	Back (%)	Chest/ Heart (%)	Eye (%)	Frost- bite (%)	Gastric (%)	Gyn (%)	Leg & Feet (%)	Mental (%)
0–25	(13)	—	7.69	—	—	15.38	—	—	15.38
26–35	(6)	—	—	—	—	—	—	—	16.67
36–45	(2)	—	—	—	—	—	—	—	—
46–55	(2)	—	—	—	—	—	—	—	—
56–65	(2)	—	—	—	—	—	—	50.00	—
66–75	(0)	—	—	—	—	—	—	—	—
76+	(2)	—	—	—	—	—	—	—	50.00
Not available	(2)	—	—	—	—	—	—	—	—

Table 19.8. Continued

| | | | | Major Complaint | | | | |
OB (%)	Respiratory (%)	Seizures (%)	Skin (%)	Substance Abuse (%)	Teeth (%)	Trauma (%)	Other (%)	Total (%)
10.71	3.57	—	3.57	3.57	—	10.71	17.86	100.02
—	3.57	—	—	3.57	7.14	3.57	21.43	100.00
12.00	—	13.00	—	13.00	—	12.00	13.00	100.00
—	—	—	—	—	—	—	33.33	99.99
—	—	—	—	—	—	—	33.33	99.99
—	—	—	—	—	—	—	—	100.00
—	—	—	—	—	—	—	—	100.00
—	—	—	—	—	—	—	—	100.00

perience reveals some of the issues a public hospital social service department may face as it reaches out to influence a community system.

The Boarding Home Project

Social Work Services has, over the years, used an informal network of boarding homes for placement of persons who need to be in a supervised environment but do not need to be placed in a nursing home.

Table 19.9. Continued

| | | | | Major Complaint | | | | |
OB (%)	Respiratory (%)	Seizures (%)	Skin (%)	Substance Abuse (%)	Teeth (%)	Trauma (%)	Other (%)	Total (%)
—	—	—	7.69	—	7.69	23.08	23.08	99.99
16.67	—	—	—	16.66	—	—	50.00	100.00
—	50.00	—	—	50.00	—	—	—	100.00
—	—	—	50.00	—	—	—	50.00	100.00
—	—	—	—	—	—	—	50.00	100.00
—	—	—	—	—	—	—	—	—
—	—	—	—	50.00	—	—	—	100.00
—	—	—	—	100.00	—	—	—	100.00

A boarding home is defined as a private residence that houses between five and fifteen people. The caretaker provides room and board, laundry, recreational activities, and assistance with personal needs such as transportation. Patients referred to a boarding home must be ambulatory without the aid of another person and must not need supervised medical care. Patients may not be placed if they have a history of violent behavior or are severely mentally retarded. Financial arrangements between the patient and provider are clarified before actual placement is made.

Boarding homes in New Orleans were not licensed when the project began. To date, the homes are not covered by Medicaid and do not meet the State Office of Family Security licensing standards for the provision of medical care. Despite the lack of licensing the boarding homes provide a placement resource that would otherwise be missing in a health care continuum of services.

The Boarding Home Team, now a component of the Patient Placement Committee, was established in August 1981. The team: (1) organizes annual visits and evaluates the conditions of the boarding homes; (2) maintains boarding home evaluation records and distributes the findings to the Social Work Services staff; (3) consults with the staff to insure that placements are made only in homes rated by the boarding home team; and (4) maintains a current listing of boarding homes.

The city originally had a law to regulate boarding homes, but it was vague and poorly enforced. As a result of input from the team and the efforts of the new boarding home association, the city has passed a new ordinance that clearly defines the role and minimum standards of boarding homes in the metropolitan area.

The Current System: Case Study of Mr. B.

The present service delivery system for homeless people at CHNO and in the New Orleans community is illustrated by the case of Mr. B., drawn from the Emergency Medical Service-Outpatient Unit files.

> Mr. B., a small, pale, fragile-looking man, age thirty-four, had walked the streets of New Orleans for five days. He had slept in abandoned buildings and on the street. He was suspicious of other street people and was unfamiliar with the shelters or soup kitchens. He had eaten out of garbage cans and was hungry. He sought help at Charity Hospital.
>
> Mr. B. was referred by the emergency room triage nurse to

Social Work Services because his complaint was hunger. A human service worker responded to the referral.

He began with reluctance to tell his story. A native of Louisiana, he had been in and out of state institutions since the age of seven. The previous month he had been discharged by court order from a mental health institution in the central part of the state. His diagnosis at discharge was mixed personality disorder with explosive and antisocial features; his medical history included diagnoses of seizure disorder and of Hodgkin's disease. Discharge plans included transportation to the town of his birth, referral to the local mental health center for support during this adjustment back into the community, and distribution of his medications. He was also instructed to go to the Social Security Office to apply for Supplemental Security Income Benefits. He was discharged with a one-week supply of drugs.

Mr. B. was a compliant patient and followed instructions. He went to the local mental health center and he applied for Social Security in the town of his birth. Two weeks later, after spending the small amount of money his father had sent him, he went to Baton Rouge and tried to get into a mental health halfway house, but did not qualify. He then traveled to New Orleans where his parents lived. They, however, did not want to support or have him live with them.

Our social worker's immediate plan was to provide Mr. B. with the basics of food, shelter, and clothing. In order to get him into a shelter for the night, she advocated on his behalf with medical staff in the emergency room to bypass the usual system so he could get clearance.

Once Mr. B. was medically cleared, one of the shelters bent its rules and allowed Mr. B. to stay until a permanent plan could be made.

Up to this point, the case management activities for Mr. B. included:

1. written and verbal requests for information from state mental health facility
2. contact with patient's family, who provided some financial resources
3. contact with three state agencies to see if Mr. B. could qualify for services
4. the filing of a reconsideration request with Social Security, since the first application was denied
5. medical services from three outpatient specialty clinics at CHNO

    6. medications purchased through CHNO Social Work Services trust funds

    7. consultation with CHNO Psychiatry Crisis Intervention Unit

    8. referral to and close collaboration with the local mental health system

Mr. B., with information and support from the social worker, negotiated the social service system. He remained compliant and followed through with referrals. His wants were simple: a safe place to call home, food, something to do, and some freedom. Mr. B. was on the waiting list for a transitional living program and attended a day treatment socialization group.

Then Mr. B.'s psychiatric condition began to deteriorate. He vacillated between guilt over crimes he had committed in the past and fantasies of prowess with guns and knives.

The system did not work quickly enough for Mr. B. He was admitted to a Charity Hospital psychiatry ward, pending admission to a state mental health institution, after he seriously threatened an employee at the day treatment program. Perhaps Mr. B. could have lived in the community if he had had access to a complete network of health care services rather than having had to piece together the fragments of a system.

Mr. B.'s case is not typical of all homeless persons who come to CHNO, but his situation is not unusual either. It does demonstrate the complexity of the service delivery system in satisfying the multiple needs of the homeless in general, and the chronically mentally ill homeless in particular.

THE IDEAL HEALTH CARE NETWORK

Representatives from the community organizations that serve the homeless in New Orleans were asked, "Where do you refer homeless people for health care services?" After a puzzled look, the common response was: "Charity Hospital, where else?" The first step necessary to develop a health care network to serve homeless people is the identification of a city's indigent health care programs, their specific admission requirements, unwritten practices, and organizational units charged with community linkage responsibilities. Major metropolitan areas throughout the country usually have a hospital, financed with public funds or operated by a religious denomination, with a mandate to serve the poor.

The second step is an accurate assessment of current organizational roles and responsibilities, identification of service delivery gaps, and conceptualization of the ideal system to deliver services to the target population.

The goal of an ideal health care system for New Orleans is to fill the current gaps in the New Orleans human service system, particularly as they relate to the chronically mentally ill homeless person, and to define an appropriate, realistic role for a public hospital whose primary purpose is acute medical care.

Primary health care and dental services would be provided at shelters or locations in the city where the homeless gather, through either on-site clinics or a mobile health care van operated by an outreach team of physician, nurse, and social worker. Immediate access to psychiatric consultation would be available.[19] Primary health care services would be vastly improved for homeless people and nonacute problems would be diverted from the public hospital's overburdened emergency rooms.

Referrals would be made to outpatient centers for more definitive tests and treatment for medical and dental needs. Transportation to and from the outpatient centers would need to be provided. The outreach health care team social worker, as case manager, would coordinate these appointments with liaison staff in the outpatient center. If the homeless person needed hospitalization, the public hospital would be contracted to provide the service.

A major gap in the current New Orleans system is absence of a place for homeless persons to stay prior to admission or for recuperation after hospitalization. There is also a chronic shortage of acute care beds for mental health and substance abuse detoxification patients.

A comprehensive emergency health care center for the homeless that would include a medical/surgical recuperative unit, a nutritional respite care unit, and a mental health and substance abuse detoxification unit is a key component of this model. The center's role would be far broader than simply providing emergency shelter for homeless persons with health-related problems.

At present, there is no single agency whose primary mission is to coordinate health care services and provide effective case management to homeless persons in New Orleans. This role would be assigned to the social work program of the comprehensive emergency health care center. The social work component's goal would be to function as case manager—to help the patient develop a long-term treatment plan that would include rehabilitation, job placement, and permanent housing. Another important role of this unit would be coordination of all formalized relationships with the other health care programs. A staff person in each network agency would collaborate closely with the social work case management unit. The agency liaison would provide on-site coordination services for the homeless and link them to the primary case manager at the comprehensive emergency health care center.

The final link in the network chain would be the development of letters of agreement between community organizations and relevant state agencies for treatment and follow-up services. The ideal health care network would provide sufficient medical care and social services to the homeless to enable as many as possible to move into stable living situations. In the presented model, the responsibility for the development and implementation of the health care network for homeless persons is assigned to a coalition composed of the agencies providing services to homeless persons.

REFERENCES

1. 1980 census of the population. General social and economic characteristics; characteristics of the population, Louisiana PC 80-1-C-20. Washington, DC: U.S. Department of Commerce, 1983; 20; 1.
2. The Office of Public Information. New Orleans: City Hall, 1984.
3. Judice V. Parish social ministry program of the Associated Catholic Charities of New Orleans. Personal interview, New Orleans, 1984.
4. Baudouin M. Emergency assistance of Associated Catholic Charities of New Orleans. Personal interview, 1984.
5. Judice V. The homeless in our midst. New Orleans: Associated Catholic Charities of New Orleans, 1984.
6. Bratton-Penny A. Office of Planning and Community Services. Letter and telephone interview. New Orleans, 1984.
7. Emergency assistance task force meeting minutes. Associated Catholic Charities of New Orleans, Inc. March 11, 1983.
8. Pitman T, Baptist Mission; Duncan J, Salvation Army; office clerk, Ozanam Inn. Telephone interviews, 1984.
9. Shelter survey: Travelers Aid Society—shelter capacity. New Orleans: Travelers Aid Society, 1984.
10. Duncan J. Salvation Army. Telephone interview, New Orleans, 1984.
11. Moreau MC. Travelers Aid Society of Greater New Orleans. Personal interview, New Orleans, 1984.
12. Fournett A. Wetmore Clinic. Telephone interview, New Orleans, 1984.
13. Lyles B. Department of Health and Human Resources, Office of Mental Health and Substance Abuse Area I memo, April 10, 1984.
14. Fossier AE. The charity hospital of Louisiana, the New Orleans medical and surgical journal. 1923.

15. Hamilton G. Hospital statistics for FY 1982–1983 and FY 1983–1984 (July–February). Telephone interview, New Orleans, 1984.
16. Staudinger M. Major emergency room/pediatric emergency room Charity Hospital at New Orleans. Personal interview, New Orleans, 1984.
17. Noya J. Walk-in clinic, Charity Hospital at New Orleans. Personal interview, New Orleans, 1984.
18. Fabre S. Emergency room, Charity Hospital at New Orleans. Personal interview, New Orleans, 1984.
19. Lutz B. City Health Department, New Orleans. Personal interview, New Orleans, 1984.

20

Health Care and the Homeless: Access to Benefits

Stephen Crystal

The two most important programs that provide access to government-paid medical care are Medicare and Medicaid. Each can, under some circumstances, be received by itself; but each is usually received in conjunction with a state or federal income-maintenance program, often without a separate application. The program most likely to be available for chronically or recently homeless individuals is Medicaid.

MEDICAID

As the successor to various forms of welfare medicine for public assistance clients, Medicaid is the principal means-tested health care benefit available to the indigent. Unlike Medicare, it essentially pays for the full cost of covered services; and although some experimental programs around the country limit the choice of medical care provider, Medicaid generally permits care by any participating provider of the client's choice, reflecting the legislative goal of avoidance of a two-tiered health care system.

Unlike Medicare, Medicaid is not a nationally uniform program. At the federal level, Medicaid legislation (Title XIX of the Social Security Act) is permissive rather than prescriptive. The federal government partially reimburses the states for medical assistance given through programs meeting federal standards for services to certain (by no means all) persons who are unable to pay for their own medical care. The amount of reimbursement varies according to a complex formula but currently is approximately half for most of the large states. In most states, the nonfederal share of the cost is borne largely or exclusively by the state.[1] In New York State, the nonfederal cost is divided between the state and county governments (city government in New York City). In the past, this cost was divided equally between state and local levels in New York. More recently, the state has moved toward a phased takeover of all Medicaid expenses, beginning with some Medicaid costs previously borne locally.

Federal financial participation is available for cases receiving one of the two major federally assisted income-maintenance benefits—Aid to Families with Dependent Children and Supplemental Security Insurance—and for some cases related to these categories that meet the family composition or disability requirements. In addition to the services provided with federal reimbursement, many states provide Medicaid benefits for individuals in need of care who do not qualify for federally assisted Medicaid benefits. While the Medically Indigent program within Medicaid permits nonrecipients of cash benefits to receive Medicaid under some circumstances, this coverage extends only to limited categories of clients. These are primarily people with very high medical expenditures resulting from extensive hospitalization or their need for long-term medical care, such as nursing home placement or home care.

The primary routes to Medicaid eligibility, therefore, are through participation in the three main income maintenance programs: Aid to Families with Dependent Children, Supplemental Security Income, and general assistance (known as Home Relief in New York State). Medicaid eligibility via the former two programs brings federal participation in the program's cost, while Medicaid to home relief recipients is entirely a state and local cost.

SUPPLEMENTARY SECURITY INCOME AND SOCIAL SECURITY DISABILITY

The federal government provides benefits to disabled persons through the Social Security Disability Insurance Program (SSD) and the Supplementary Security Income Program (SSI). Under both statutes, *disability* is defined as "the inability to engage in any substantial gainful activity by reason of any medically determinable physical or mental impairment which can be expected to result in death or which has lasted or can be expected to last for a continuous period of not less than twelve months." [42 U.S.C. 423(d)(1)(A), 1382c(a)(3)(A)]. An individual "shall be determined to be under a disability only if his physical or mental impairment or impairments are of such severity that he is not only unable to do his previous work but cannot, considering his age, education, and work experience, engage in any other kind of substantial gainful work which exists in the national economy" [42 U.S.C. 423 (d)(2) (A), 1382c(a)(3)(B)].

Interpretation of the statute by the Social Security Administration (SSA) in the last several years, particularly with respect to mental disability, has been extremely severe—to an extent that has been criticized by a number of federal courts as going well beyond what is authorized in law. Testimony in 1983 congressional hearings included scores of horror stories in which clearly grossly disabled individuals were denied benefits by SSA administrative staff. As many as 50 percent of denials by administrative staff were overturned on appeal by hearing officers (administrative law judges). Even though significant liberalization has taken place under congressional and court prodding, it remains important for those who help the homeless secure benefits to understand that eligibility determination is a multistage process and that unfavorable administrative determinations can often be reversed at a later stage. Thus, carrying cases through to appeal can often secure initially denied benefits. Social Security Administration staff routinely advise claimants that representation by counsel is unnecessary and will not affect the results; but this advice may not be in the interest of the client. Expert representation, whether legal or otherwise, can often win a benefit that would otherwise be denied. Thus, a major service that programs can provide to the homeless is assistance in securing SSI benefits (and the accompanying Medicaid eligibility). Important elements in this assistance include arranging for appropriate medical examinations and securing appropriate written evaluations for submission to the Social Security Administration.

By regulation, SSA has adopted a five-step sequential evaluation process to determine eligibility for SSI and SSD benefits. While these programs are completely federally financed, with relatively uniform national guidelines for eligibility and benefits, eligibility determination is performed by state offices.

The procedure in New York State is comparable to that in most other states. Initial disability determinations are made by the New York State Office of Disability Determinations (State ODD) pursuant to a contract between the state and the SSA. The case record on any claim is compiled by a lay disability analyst, who gathers substantiating information or, where such information is insufficient, procures one or more medical or psychiatric examinations. Assessments of psychiatric disability are based on a review of this file by a staff physician employed by State ODD. This assessment is referred back to a disability analyst or specialist, a State ODD employee. After considering the claimant's residual functional capacity, age, experience, and education, this person decides whether the claimant can be expected to return to his former work or to engage in any other substantial gainful activity.

All decisions by the State ODD are subject to a Quality Assurance Review by the regional and central offices of SSA. The central office similarly reviews the performance of SSA regional offices (Tier III review). The standards reflected in these reviews constitute de facto eligibility standards that are not necessarily based on statute, as many courts have found. A large number of returns from a higher level causes the regional and state administrations to pressure the review physicians to conform to the federal line from Baltimore. Ultimately, the potential threat exists of contract termination for state offices that do not follow administratively determined eligibility policies to the SSA's satisfaction.

SSI is extremely valuable to the homeless; it enables them to receive monthly checks to establish their own households or to pay the cost of family homes, adult homes, or other licensed residences where their special needs can be met. It also gives them categorical eligibility for Medicaid. Federal enabling statutes originally barred residents of public institutions from receiving SSI. This bar was intended to prevent the federal government from assuming large new expenses for residents of state mental hospitals and prisons. However, since May 1983, partly as a result of advocacy by New York City and other cities concerned with caring for the homeless, SSI eligibles are permitted three months of benefits in any twelve-month period of residence in a public emergency shelter. This affords them the opportunity to prepare for a smooth transition from the shelter into an independent living setting without waiting to have benefits reactivated.

HRA's Shelter Outreach Project

Because SSI is such a valuable link to other services to the homeless, particularly health services, the New York City Human Resources Administration (HRA) makes a concerted effort to assist shelter residents to apply for SSI through its Shelter Outreach Project. Shelter staff screen the residents to determine which have a history of SSI receipt, application, or rejection. Staff preselect residents who are likely to meet the requirements, complete SSI applications, and prepare documentation and background material. Shelter staff arrange for medical examinations and prepare the resident for visits from HRA, the State Office of Disability Determinations, and SSA teams. This approach offers a significant model that can help address the logistical problems of coordinating medical examinations and eligibility interviews on behalf of clients who are mentally ill, confused, and have difficulty negotiating bureaucratic systems.

However, the severe administrative standards for eligibility imposed by SSA have limited success rates, even for carefully selected clients. Initial results from this SSI Shelter Outreach Project were disheartening. Approximately 80 percent of the applications were initially rejected. All rejections were appealed. Between November 1981 and August 1982, of 258 persons assisted by the Shelter Outreach teams, only 103 had been accepted for benefits, of whom 42 were former recipients who were reinstated. Since the inception of the program, the acceptance rate has improved to about 47 percent. Some slackening of standards, as a result of judicial and congressional pressure, as well as experience with the program, has helped to improve success rates, and the Shelter Outreach Project continues to link homeless persons to SSI benefits, projecting 300 successful applications in fiscal year 1985.

HRA has recently contracted for legal services to help clients obtain benefits or regain them if they were improperly terminated. This approach of contracting for expert legal assistance and advocacy in the disability determination process may be applicable in a variety of situations, since the process can be complex; many local legal services organizations have acquired substantial experience in handling these cases because of the large number of redeterminations initiated by SSA during the past several years.

Despite considerable effort to make the application process as efficient as possible and to reduce the stress on the applicant, HRA found that restrictive interpretations of SSA regulations deprived a large number of mentally ill homeless people of benefits. Denial of SSI to a mentally ill person means more than not receiving a monthly check; to many, it means a severe medical setback and roadblock to other services, such as Medicaid or an adult home, and probable delay in moving from a shelter to a more independent environment.

SSI in Transition

As of mid-1984, SSI eligibility constituted a patchwork situation in transition. Most of the twelve federal Courts of Appeals had rejected one or more of the administrative standards for disability, particularly with respect to mental disability. Contrary to usual practice, these adverse decisions had not been translated into general practice, even in the circuits in which the decision was handed down—a pattern sharply criticized by a number of federal judges. Congressional action was receiving consideration. In such a situation, the advocacy role, as well as the individual client representation role of programs for the homeless, takes on particular importance; maintaining current knowledge of practices is also important. Despite the problems, SSI offers the best opportunity to secure for a mentally ill or physically disabled homeless person a benefit that is relatively permanent; provides the basis, with state supplementation for which recipients are eligible, to finance adult home or family home care; and brings with it Medicaid benefits.

Some individuals may be qualified for SSI or Social Security benefits, particularly on the grounds of mental disability, but have difficulty in handling funds provided to them. Social Security laws and regulations permit the appointment of a representative payee in such cases; in fact, a representative payee is required by regulation for alcoholics and drug addicts receiving SSI, though this provision is often unenforced. Shelters or other programs for the homeless can apply to be named as representative payee for a client; they can then receive the client's check and expend the funds on his or her behalf.[2]

MEDICARE

Medicare is a nationally uniform program, primarily for the elderly, administered directly by the federal government through the Social Security Administration, whose district offices are the point of application. It provides for partial payment of hospital, physician, and some other covered services, primarily for individuals who are in receipt of Social Security retirement benefits. Some very limited categories of recipients, such as end-stage renal failure patients and recipients of Social Security disability after a waiting period, have also been made eligible for benefits.

Substantial copayments and deductibles under Medicare, as well as coverage limitations, restrict its usefulness for homeless individuals without another significant source of income. Part A, which covers hospitalization, requires a deductible of $356 for each hospital stay beginning in 1984. Part B, covering physician and some other services, requires a premium of $14 per month and an annual deductible of $75, as well as a 20 percent copayment for services used. Because of these requirements, as well as coverage limitations, Medicare covers only 45 percent of the participants' health care costs.

Medicare is relevant to only a small part of the homeless population, because it is primarily a program for the elderly. However, it can be an important resource for elderly homeless individuals, and securing any Social Security benefits a client may be entitled to is particularly important because of the value of concomitant Medicare coverage.

Elderly homeless individuals without substantial Social Security checks or other income may be eligible for the Old Age category of SSI, which does not require a disability test. This brings the more valuable Medicaid benefits as well as Medicare.

PUBLIC ASSISTANCE

The homeless with children may be eligible for Aid to Families with Dependent Children. This brings with it Medicaid eligibility as well as possible eligibility for emergency housing services. The public assistance programs for which homeless adult individuals are likely to qualify are the general assistance programs. However, these programs have been severely restricted or eliminated in a number of states, in a trend with ominous implications for the homeless.

New York and a number of other states provide full Medicaid benefits to general assistance/home relief recipients, at state and local expense. New York City has made special arrangements for expedited handling of referrals from shelter to income-maintenance centers. From July 1, 1982, through January 31, 1984, 3484 persons were accepted for public assistance, thus receiving Medicaid eligibility as well. Special referral and processing arrangements between shelters and income-maintenance offices thus offer an important means for providing not only the financial means for community living but also access to health care on an ongoing basis.

HEALTH CARE FOR THE HOMELESS
IN SHELTERS

In operating what is by far the largest system of public shelters in the nation, New York City encountered the need to provide health services to shelter residents and has developed a network to provide such care. The three-tier model includes primary care clinics in public shelters, referrals to clinics at backup hospitals for more specialized care, and a special procedure that makes longer-term shelter clients eligible for Medicaid without normal processing and documentation requirements.

In-Shelter Services

At a number of the City shelters, on-site medical clinics provide primary care. Physicians, nurses, and/or nurse practitioners examine all shelter residents who request medical care or who are referred by shelter staffs. These clinics provide referrals to backup hospitals for needed outpatient or inpatient care that is beyond their capacity to provide.

The City funds similar clinics at storefront outreach centers, which is an important way of bringing care and services to those homeless persons who are reluctant to come into regular shelters and might not otherwise receive care. Outreach centers provide basic health care and screening in a setting that is more reassuring than a hospital or shelter clinic would be.

Clinic Referrals

Through special financial arrangements, the City reimburses backup hospitals for outpatient clinic services provided to patients referred from City shelters and outreach centers. This arrangement provides financing for what otherwise would be nonreimbursable services given by the hospital to homeless individuals.

Medicaid

Clients in New York City shelters qualify for Medicaid benefits after spending fifteen days in a shelter. Eligibility is granted for ninety days and may be recertified for additional ninety-day periods as long as the client remains in the shelter system. Through regulations issued by New York City, those with special needs that cannot be met by on-site clinics may immediately register for Medicaid, even before spending fifteen days in the system.

PROGRAMS FOR THE HOMELESS AS ADVOCATES FOR BENEFITS

Working to secure benefits for the mentally impaired homeless in particular can have much the quality of the original Catch-22. Nevertheless, working with the homeless to secure entitlements is among the most important services that can be provided by programs serving them. Arrangements for access to SSI, Medicaid, and other benefits constitute the chief route to health care, as well as to attaining more independent, stable living arrangements.

REFERENCES

1. Medicaid/Medicare Management Institute. Data on the Medicaid program: eligibility, services, expenditures. Baltimore: Health Care Financing Administration, 1979.
2. Project Focus. Representative payee: questions and answers for caseworkers. New York: New York City Human Resources Administration, 1982. Available from Project Focus, HRA, 60 Hudson Street, 9th Floor, New York, New York 10013, at no charge.

PART V

VIABLE MODELS

21

Boston, Massachusetts: The Pine Street Inn Nurses' Clinic and Tuberculosis Program

Eileen Reilly and Barbara N. McInnis

I. OVERVIEW OF THE PINE STREET INN BY EILEEN REILLY

The Pine Street Inn is an emergency shelter for the homeless, located in Boston's South End. The Inn has 300 beds for men and fifty for women. In cold weather, after the beds are filled, an additional 250 men and women sleep in the lobbies on benches and on the floor.

PINE STREET'S SERVICES AND ATTITUDE

A nurses' clinic is conducted in the shelter every evening, including weekends, and serves approximately seventy patients in the men's clinic and twenty-five in the women's clinic. The goal of the clinic is to help the guests maintain optimal health, given the conditions of life that they face. Special effort has been made to identify and treat homeless persons afflicted with tuberculosis. This program is detailed later in the chapter.

The clinic was started in April 1972 by a group of nurses from Boston City Hospital who had become increasingly aware of the special needs of the Pine Street guests. The nurses saw the men (Pine Street did not serve women until 1980) discharged from the hospital with instructions they were unable to carry out, prescriptions they could not pay for, and appointments they most likely would not keep. Typically, a homeless man with a leg ulcer, for example, would have no place to rest, no water available to soak his leg, and no access to proper nourishment. For various reasons, he would be unable or unwilling to go to an outpatient clinic for daily dressing changes; his bottle of antibiotics, if he had been able to obtain a social worker voucher to receive them, would be lost or stolen on the street. In a few weeks he would return to the hospital with a serious infection and would need to be admitted.

With the encouragement of Paul Sullivan, who was then the Inn's director, the nurses decided to come to Pine Street for a month to study the health needs of the guests, intending to let the guests identify their own needs.[1] After a month's time it was determined that the needs of the guests were indeed appropriate for nursing intervention, and thus the independent nurses' clinic was founded.

The services offered include triage and referral of the guests to the appropriate agency; helping guests identify their health problems and seek help before a crisis; helping them with treatments they would normally do at home if their living situation permitted; providing first aid; and holding medication for the guest, administering one day's supply at a time.

The clinic began with all volunteer personnel. Presently, we have four full-time staff paid by Pine Street, a public health nurse who works for Boston Health and Hospitals, and two psychiatric nurses assigned to Pine Street by the Massachusetts Department of Mental Health—one who works full-time and the other, part-time.

The addition of psychiatric nurses was in response to the increasing number of deinstitutionalized mental patients seen. These nurses identify the deinstitutionalized, intervene in crises, and help the staff deal with guests who have psychiatric problems. The nurses are present to be advocates, to facilitate entry into the hospital when guests need intervention, and to work as liaisons to the Department of Mental Health. Nobody is forced into treatment.

We have two full-time coordinators, one for each clinic. They are responsible for follow-up, making appointments for the guests, recording information on charts, and arranging for volunteers to accompany the guests to the hospital. My role as administrator includes outreaching to the hospitals to which we refer people, working with emergency room personnel, and coordinating the volunteer program for the clinic. The full-time nurse assures continuity of care for the guests, communicates with doctors and nurses who treat the guests at the hospital, and gives direct nursing care. She also educates the staff and volunteers: she speaks at staff meetings on such subjects as seizures or hypothermia and teaches the counselors when to call an ambulance.

The most common ailments that the guests present include respiratory diseases, such as pneumonia, tuberculosis, and bronchitis; scabies and lice; stasis ulcers; hypertension; cardiac disorders; seizures; frostbite and hypothermia; and gynecological problems. Many of their afflictions are caused or exacerbated by alcoholism, mental illness, exposure, malnutrition, exhaustion, and crowded living conditions. Health problems in the homeless are also complicated by their alienation and estrangement. Many have lost touch with their families and friends and have no one to encourage or help them.

Because homeless people often use emergency rooms for shelter, hospital staff often assume that they are not there for legitimate medical reasons. This attitude and practice prevents access to health care. In addition, homeless people are often unable to negotiate their way through the hospital bureaucracy.

Serious health problems are often neglected because the homeless person struggles merely to survive. For the person on the street, a broken bone may go untreated because of more immediate needs for shelter, food, and community. Even more significant are the despair and feelings of worthlessness that prevent them from caring about their injury or sickness.

We believe that the first task of the Pine Street Inn nurses' clinic is to respect and value the dignity of each individual. The philosophy of Pine Street holds that the most basic need of guests is to be accepted for who they are; that the real work at the shelter is not simply to provide a bed, food, clothing, and health care but to welcome those who are otherwise outcast and to call them by their names. In this way, staff and volunteers create an atmosphere of trust and caring, making the clinic a place where guests do not feel threatened or judged.

Emphasis is placed on gradually developing relationships, using a one-to-one approach. For example, one guest, Frank, was becoming increasingly ill and losing weight but would not seek medical attention because of his alienation and psychosis. There was a counselor at Pine Street who would search for him, find him, and sit with him each day. In the evening someone would invite him into the clinic. After several weeks, he finally began to come to the door of the clinic and eventually would come inside and accept some juice. When he finally agreed to go to the hospital, he was found to have intestinal cancer.

Or take the example of foot soaks. Clinic staff give many of them—they are therapeutic for ulcers, callouses, and blisters. But some foot soaks are instrumental in developing relationships. Some of the psychotic women will not address their problems of hypertension but will come in to soak their feet. These foot soaks thus become starting points for knowing and working with some guests.

PINE STREET'S SUCCESS

Another factor that contributes to the clinic's success is its accessibility. Located within the shelter, the clinic is open while bed tickets, clothing, and supper are given out. It is easy to use the clinic: a guest simply gives a name. It does not even have to be the real name. An attempt is made to get a data base, such as next-of-kin and major health problems; but if people are unable or unwilling to give information, they still receive treatment.

Follow-up and continuity help to make the clinic succeed. We keep track of appointments and remind the guests of them. We maintain a daily call list of people who need to be reminded to come in, and the coordinators look for them in the lobbies and the park after supper. The coordinators or nurses often call the hospital to find out a guest's treatment plan. We also have written referral forms that we complete on all people who go to the hospital, whether to the emergency room or to an outpatient clinic. These referrals contain the specifics regarding the request for evaluation, along with any pertinent history we might have. We request that the doctor or nurse who sees the person return a written treatment plan at the bottom of our referral sheet. Charts are kept on each person, as well as a medication card, which enhances continuity and is helpful for other agencies, such as detoxes and hospitals, that call Pine Street for information.

Our relationship to nearby hospitals, particularly Boston City Hospital and New England Medical Center, is significant. Ongoing meetings take place between Pine Street clinic staff and emergency room doctors and nurses, emergency medical technicians, social workers, and hospital security. We invite them to come for tours of Pine Street, and all nurses who start work at Boston City Hospital hear about Pine Street during their orientation. We speak to nursing and medical students about the problems of homeless persons, for the sake of educating, changing attitudes, and recruiting volunteers.

It is not only the clinic at Pine Street that has an effect on the health of the guests. Our transportation service provides five trips throughout the day and night to local hospitals, and two daily trips to a detox. Malnutrition has decreased because of the Inn's food program. Two meals are provided daily; volunteer groups donate the evening meal.

We have a hot room in the shower area where the guests' clothing is placed each night. High temperatures kill whatever lice or mites may be on the clothing.

The Inn's counseling staff is sensitive to and knowledgeable about health problems. They make referrals to hospitals, detoxes, and nursing homes; they know how to recognize and treat infestations, and how to give first aid for seizures, trauma, and cardiac problems.

Since the move to a new site in 1980, we have been able to provide a more healthy environment for the guests, with improved air circulation, cleaning and maintenance of the building, and more space for each guest.

The volunteer program of the nurses' clinic is of utmost value. Volunteers come with warmth and enthusiasm, as well as a variety of skills. People with varied backgrounds—such as a retired postal worker, a school teacher, and students—volunteer as clinic receptionists. Nursing and medical students provide services under the direction of a nurse. Nursing students from local colleges work in the clinic for an entire semester and choose one client to work with closely.

After years of working at Pine Street, all who work there—staff and volunteers—feel that what they receive from the guests is far greater than what they give. The results of the clinic's tuberculosis program is but one example of the intangible rewards that work with the homeless brings, beyond the walls of the Pine Street Inn and into the community at large.

II. THE TUBERCULOSIS PROGRAM
BY BARBARA N. McINNIS

In 1970 I made my first visit to the Pine Street Inn as a public health district nurse, looking for tuberculosis (TB) patients assigned to me for follow-up. I walked into the Inn and was shocked and frightened by what I saw: a large number of dirty, drunken, and sometimes disoriented men crowded into a dimly lit lobby. Some were standing; others sat on benches; many were lying on the floor with bags, bits of food and newspapers strewn about them. Everything and everyone was enveloped in a haze of cigarette smoke. I hurried through, into the director's office and out a side door, pausing only to give a lobby counselor a list of patients I was looking for; I never looked back.

In the following days I would get an occasional call from the Inn saying that someone from the list had been found. I would make arrangements for that person to go to the TB Clinic at the South End Health Unit (SEHU). In 1971 this list became a "Lost to Care List" and eventually became known as the TB "Wanted List." My working hours in those days were 9:00 A.M. to 5:00 P.M., so I began making visits to the Pine Street Inn in the early afternoon. However, the majority of men did not appear at the Inn until 4:00 P.M.; my success at locating people on the Wanted List was very low.

In April of 1972 the Volunteer Nurses' Clinic was started at Pine Street Inn (PSI) by a group of nurses from the Boston City Hospital. I began to receive telephone calls from the clinic nurses about some of the patients I had been looking for. The nurses had, for instance, spoken to an Inn guest and motivated him to go to the TB clinic. One of the nurses even accompanied the men to be sure they arrived at the clinic. In a study done in the clinic's first month, 193 men were seen, 2 complained of current TB symptoms, and 12 gave a history of treatment for active TB. Half of this group "thought they were over it"[1] but had doubts. Some of the men had left the sanitorium early, had not received final checkups and chest x-rays, or had taken their medication sporadically.

After several months of calls from the PSI clinic nurses, I became embarrassed because they were finding the patients I had been looking for. In July of 1972 I volunteered in the nurses' clinic at the Pine Street Inn. I have been there ever since.

GENESIS OF THE PROGRAM

Two studies done in 1972 brought the PSI tuberculosis problem to the fore. The Pisarcik study was cited previously; the second study tried to match the names of recalcitrant patients with active TB to men who had stayed one or more nights at PSI.[2] The data were obtained from a PSI card file that listed the name, date, place of birth, and medical history—information that each guest volunteered on his first night at the shelter.

In this study many of the men were listed as "chronic nonresidents," but the data cards indicated that 60 percent had been born in Massachusetts and 58 percent of that number had been born in Boston. Therefore, the TB patients at PSI previously considered nonresidents were in large part natives of the city or state. Most had not moved very far.

A chronic nonresident as defined by Massachusetts General Law (chap. 111, sect. 80) is a person who evidences in past history an inability or unwillingness to establish and maintain a stable residence. This instability, and the generally poor living standard that results, exposes the person and others to infection and makes them a special problem for tuberculosis disease control.

Several letters were exchanged between the Pine Street Inn and the appropriate city and state agencies regarding the TB problem. A proposal was drawn up, and out of it emerged a position for a full-time public health nurse and a weekly TB clinic at PSI. The purposes of this new TB program were to provide intensive and continuous health services to a high-risk TB group within a street-based population and to insure that whatever medical treatment was ordered would be carried out.

In May 1973 a full-time public health nurse began working at PSI. Her role was, and continues to be, to relate to the homeless guests of the Inn as a friend rather than as a representative of the establishment. Her goal is to get those persons with tuberculosis into treatment. Symptomatic guests are screened by use of the Mantoux test and chest x-rays. The TB clinic physician performs the medical evaluation; the Massachusetts Department of Public Health provides free medication. Hospital referrals are made when a person is gravely ill or sputum smears are positive for acid-fast bacilli. Mantoux testing is also done every six months for staff.

In September 1973 the Pine Street Inn TB Clinic was staffed by a physician and clerk one night per week. An x-ray technician and clerk to take chest x-rays were on the premises two nights per week.

OPERATION OF THE PROGRAM

In 1974 there were four deaths among the PSI guests due to active tuberculosis. We found many cases among a population that previously seemed impossible to locate. Those with positive skin tests were given chest x-rays when possible. Follow-up was limited because of the lifestyle of the alcoholic street person.

Between 1971 and 1975 we used the Menace Law for those guests who had positive AFB smears. These same men were sleeping in a room with 90 to 110 others, drinking out of the same bottles on the street, and living in generally poor conditions. Some of the staff also contracted tuberculosis during those early years, but since 1980 none has.

The Menace Law—under sections 94A and 94C, chapter 111 of the General Laws of Massachusetts—allows a person to be removed from the home or street and placed into a medical treatment facility if, first, the person has verified TB; second, the person is unwilling or unable to accept proper medical treatment; and third, the person poses a serious danger to the health of the local community. Only after all the legal procedures are completed and adequate proof provided may the person be remanded to a TB sanitorium.

In 1978 a typical case study was that of Mr. W. B., aged sixty, who slept on the lobby floor of PSI, was cachectic, coughed up large amounts of sputum, was feverish, and perspired profusely. He seldom ate a meal, but chain smoked. He was a paranoid schizophrenic whose delusions led him to believe that the x-ray machine was a hostile animal of impending doom. He was gravely ill but conscious. There was no way we could convince him to go to the hospital. We could not employ the Menace Law because we did not have a documented positive sputum or an abnormal chest x-ray. He was dying before our eyes.

Finally, one of the counselors convinced him to go to a hospital. The hospital doctor said the man was paranoid, just needed some food, and should return to the shelter and eat. The doctor ignored what we wrote on the referral about W.B., his symptoms and history. W.B. returned to the shelter, to an upset but helpless staff. Three days later, he lost consciousness and was taken by ambulance to another hospital. He was admitted, diagnosed, and died three days later of active tuberculosis.

Since then, conditions have improved considerably. The Pine Street Inn moved into a new building in 1980; the staff was increased, and ongoing education keeps them aware of the symptoms and conditions of a potential tuberculosis case. The clinic can then follow up at an early stage with people who might not otherwise be seen. Over the years the guests have developed a close and trusting relationship with the clinic to the extent that they want a chest x-ray every time they develop a cough.

The clinic's cost to the city in 1983 was $5000 for the physician's services; its cost to the state was $53,460 for the services of the x-ray technician, two clerks, and one nurse.

When we were preparing to move into our new building in 1980, we encountered a lot of community opposition from people who feared their children would contract TB from wine bottles the guests left on the street. This fear was increased when an article from a clinical research magazine published in 1974 suddenly appeared in the community in 1980. A doctor from Harvard University had listed the census tract where the Pine Street Inn was located as having 294 cases of tu-

Table 21.1.   Active Cases of and Deaths from Tuberculosis

	Cases of Active TB:			Deaths from TB:	
Year	Mass.	Boston	PSI*	Boston	PSI
1967		276	8		
1969		275	13**	36	
1970		308	26	36	
1971	763	299	41***	26	
1974	650	220	18	13	4
1978	580	170	5		2
1982	503	150	3		0
1983	389	137	2		0

*Pine Street Inn.

**Increase due to new management at Pine Street Inn.

***Boston Alcohol Detoxification Project began its services in the basement of the Pine Street Inn, June 1971.

berculosis per 100,000 population, the highest in the country at that time.[3]

Table 21.1 lists active cases of tuberculosis and deaths from tuberculosis and is made available from the Massachusetts Department of Public Health Statistics. Where no number is given, data were unavailable.

In 1974 we had ninety-two men receiving isoniazid (INH); today we have three individuals taking INH. There have been no cases of active tuberculosis found among the more than fifty nightly female guests since the women's unit opened in 1980.

REFERENCES

1. Pisarcik G. The health needs of the Pine Street community: a study. Unpublished study, April 1972.
2. Cremone J. A study of tuberculosis for the Massachusetts Department of Public Health. Unpublished study, 1972.
3. Broderick A, Watson A, Simmons G, LaForce M, Huber G. Consumption in skid row: a perspective on the focality of active tuberculosis in an urban center. Unpublished study, Tufts University School of Medicine, 1974.

22

New York City:
The Saint Vincent's Hospital
SRO and Shelter Programs

Barbara Conanan and Mary Jean O'Brien

Saint Vincent's Hospital and Medical Center of New York has provided health care to single-room-occupancy (SRO) residents and homeless people since 1969.

The original concept for our program developed from an intern's[1-3] observations in the emergency room. He noted that a number of men who arrived by ambulance were moribund or dead and recognized that many of these people resided at the same address, a place called the Greenwich Hotel at 160 Bleecker Street in New York (see Chapter 1).

During the eighteen months in which we ran a free clinic at the hotel, among the common causes of complaint was trauma inflicted by other residents of the hotel.[2,3]

Many residents were extremely ill and had myriad medical and psychosocial problems; they were the sickest, the tip of the iceberg. Another segment would not use the emergency room; they elected to remain in their hotel rooms to die.

After the hotel was closed down, many of the men were placed into the string of SROs along the West Side of Manhattan.

We subsequently took our staff, experience, and motivation into the smaller SROs. We now work in eleven of them, along the lower West Side and in the Times Square area.

SROs

Single-room-occupancies function and advertise as hotels, and charge at least $50 per week for a room. More realistically, the minimum payment is $75 per week and is increasing.[6] The room is usually 5 feet by 8 feet; the landlord provides a cot and dresser.

Hotels are regularly in disrepair. Services and facilities are limited: common bathrooms have only cold running water and malfunctioning plumbing; there are no kitchen facilities.[5]

Three distinct groups reside in SRO hotels: those who have special problems, such as alcoholism and drug abuse; the working poor, the retired and fragile elderly, the physically handicapped, the mentally disabled, and those who can afford only inexpensive housing; and families, mostly mothers with young children.[4,5] Many are disaffiliated from family, religious institutions, friends, and community. They exist marginally on public assistance or social security income.[5] (See Table 22.1.)

Teams of nurses and social workers go to the hotels on regular schedules, once a week, twice a week, or as need dictates to provide health screening, physical examinations, treatment of minor medical problems, and medical referral. Physicians are available for emergencies or for specific problems that require medical opinion.

PROVIDING ON-SITE CARE

The teams provide needed services that fall into several broad categories.

Case Finding

In an attempt to find cases, health providers need to know the hotel system and how it works. An amicable relationship should be established with hotel management, who can provide rosters with the names of residents and their room numbers. The team can then aggressively seek residents by knocking on doors and introducing themselves. If residents are unavailable, a note is left informing them of the team's

Table 22.1. Demographic and Clinical Data from Four SROs

Category	Barbour	Jane West	Keller	New Holland
Total population	121	181	88	35
Male	109 (90%)	156 (86%)	82 (93%)	29 (85%)
Female	12 (10%)	25 (14%)	6 (7%)	6 (16%)
Alcoholics	48 (40%)	37 (20%)	21 (24%)	12 (33%)
Psychiatric patients	18 (15%)	42 (23%)	28 (32%)	12 (33%)
Drug abusers	37 (30%)	2 (1%)	17 (19%)	2 (6%)
Ex-offenders	55 (45%)	18 (10%)	10 (11%)	1 (3%)
Physically Handicapped	11 (9%)	3 (2%)	12 (14%)	2 (6%)
Multiply Handicapped	1 (1%)	0 (0%)	10 (11%)	0 (0%)
60 years of age or older with psychiatric problem	3 (2%)	14 (8%)	7 (8%)	2 (6%)
Medical or psychiatric history unknown	103 (85%)	14 (8%)	0 (0%)	5 (15%)
P.A. Clients	93 (77%)	99 (55%)	41 (47%)	10 (28%)
SSI-OAA	6 (5%)	21 (12%)	12 (14%)	1 (3%)
SSI-AD	11 (9%)	2 (29%)	31 (35%)	10 (28%)
SSI-AB	0 (0%)	2 (1%)	0 (0%)	0 (0%)
Income unknown	0 (0%)	0 (0%)	0 (0%)	0 (0%)
Employment income	11 (9%)	4 (2%)	3 (3%)	3 (8%)
Other income	0 (0%)	3 (2%)	1 (1%)	0 (0%)
Ethnicity				
Black	60 (50%)	76 (42%)	30 (34%)	10 (28%)
Hispanic	22 (18%)	23 (13%)	13 (15%)	3 (8%)
White	36 (30%)	81 (45%)	43 (49%)	20 (56%)
Other	3 (2%)	1 (0.5%)	2 (2%)	2 (6%)
Age				
18–25	6 (5%)	18 (10%)	2 (2%)	2 (6%)
26–40	72 (60%)	41 (23%)	38 (43%)	10 (28%)
41–60	36 (30%)	83 (46%)	36 (41%)	13 (35%)
61+	7 (5%)	39 (21%)	12 (14%)	10 (28%)

attempt to reach them and the time of their next visit. Residents who act as gatekeepers can be a valuable resource to the caregiver, as well as provide social interaction with residents who may be in the lobby.

Health providers need to recognize that rooms in an SRO hotel are the residents' homes. Professionals must respect the need for residents' privacy, as well as the desire to be left alone. Systems are developed that inform residents of the team's availability and give the residents some control over medical intervention and "future meddling" in their lives by the team.

Medical Team Intervention

Our experience indicates that residents gradually become amenable to intervention when the need arises. They are more receptive because in many cases relationships have been established through the team's honesty, constancy, persistence, persuasiveness, and sense of humor in the face of many rejecting and resisting encounters. Trust begins when the residents realize that the team accepts them on whatever level they function.

Many professionals feel very uncomfortable in an uncontrolled environment that is filled with unpredictability and people unamenable and sometimes hostile toward assistance. The result could be mutual alienation, fear, and mistrust. Therefore, one must realize and remember that many of these people have been deprived and that their feelings and behavior are defense mechanisms designed to push people away because of previous painful experiences. Professionals must share a *part* of themselves to people who are exposing *all* of themselves.

The team works constantly at problem solving and creating practical and realistic medical and social services for the residents. Getting these people to accept and maintain treatment on an ongoing basis can be tedious, laborious, and frustrating, but with occasional rewards. We at St. Vincent's have found that it is the process and interaction with the patients themselves that is rewarding. Notions of success need to be modified to acknowledge seemingly small effects which, when accumulated over time, can change lives.

Once a resident is amenable to intervention, there are several steps that are performed in the hotel:

1. Identification of the problems of the individuals (medical, surgical, nutritional, or psychosocial).
2. Medical examination and/or physical assessment. A medical history is requested. Vital signs should be obtained on the first visit.
3. Treatment, such as dressing changes, suture removal, and so forth.
4. Diagnostic studies. Procedures such as blood work and electrocardiograms can occasionally be done on-site. However, residents are encouraged to attend the outpatient department for all diagnostic testing so that they can begin using the health care system effectively.
5. Monitoring of medication and determination of whether residents fully understand the directions. If the staff suspect patients are

not regularly taking their medication, they should confront the patients in a nonthreatening manner. This is important for follow-up fostering of compliance.

6. Monitoring of vital signs. This is done to detect a wide range of medical problems (such as cardiac disease, hypertension, diabetes mellitus), to determine side effects of medications, and to learn if patients are benefiting from the prescribed treatment regime.

Monitoring Appointments

The importance of other problems in the resident's life may override clinic appointments; for many health care is not a priority. Therefore, residents have to be reminded constantly of clinic appointments and scheduled diagnostic testing.

Counseling and Education

These services are tailored to the individuals' particular medical problems or psychosocial needs.

Referral

SRO residents often have to be referred to other facilities for care, detoxification, family planning, or dental work. Follow-up on referral to subspecialty clinics and dieticians is necessary.

Social Service

Social workers are the ombudsmen and advocates. They act as liaisons and transporters and help residents secure or maintain entitlements.

Hospitalization

Patients are visited when they are hospitalized. On occasion, if a patient is not hospitalized at Saint Vincent's Hospital (SVH), we will visit them at other hospitals. Telephone contact is maintained between house staff and outreach staff to ensure follow-up after discharge.

SHELTERS

In 1969, in addition to the SRO health care program, Saint Vincent's Hospital began to provide medical services to the Men's Shelter on the Lower East Side. The hospital also provided medical backup support for a freestanding alcoholism detoxification unit, the Manhattan Bowery Corporation. Due to property tax abatement incentives, SRO hotel closings, low-cost housing shortages, and budget cuts, more people had been forced onto the streets. We are currently running clinics at four shelter sites. While some SROs are atrocious dwellings, they do provide housing, a private room, stability, and a secure environment. Shelters were never meant to be permanent housing, but for many they are the only alternative to the streets.[7]

The four shelters in which our teams work are as follows:

1. New York City Municipal Men's Shelter at 8 East 3rd Street.

This shelter is located in the Bowery area of Manhattan, on New York's skid row. It functions seven days a week as the clearing center for most of the city's other shelters. This unit itself does not provide housing, but instead arranges for placement elsewhere of about 6000 men each night. Three meals a day are served. Our clinic in the building functions forty hours each week, staffed by a physician, nurse, and corpsman. About 1200 individual patients are seen each year, with 5000 visits. Twenty thousand records have been accumulated since 1969.

2. Charles Gay Shelter, Keener Building, Wards Island (in the East River).

This shelter houses about 850 men and provides meals and clothing. Housing is dormitory style, and each person is given a foot locker. A substantial number of residents seem to perceive this place as a permanent residence.

Our clinic is in operation seven days for sixty hours each week. Three nurses, one physician, and two male aides make up the staff. Lab specimens and electrocardiograms are obtained on site and brought to Saint Vincent's Hospital for processing. We record over 10,000 patient contacts each year.

3. West Side Cluster—Antonio Olivieri Center—West 30th Street, Manhattan.

This unit, a store front drop-in center run by a voluntary agency, is for women only. By regulation, beds and cots are not allowed. About 69 women, 25 percent of whom are long stayers, are present each night, sleeping on chairs. Food, clothing, and bathing facilities are offered.

Our nurse–physician–social worker team is present nineteen hours a week. Because there are markedly high indices of psychosis in this group of patients, much of our time and attention is devoted to establishing trust. We carry out any form of direct health service that our patients will allow. Over the years since 1981, when we started work at the Cluster, the patients have gradually grown more trusting, even though it may still take several months to complete a physical examination. We now have about sixty patient contacts a week.

4. First Moravian Church—Coffee Pot Program—Lexington Avenue and 30th Street, Manhattan.

This program runs a drop-in center for men and women. Meals, shower facilities, and clothing are available. About 125 people are seen during the day; and approximately 10 sleep on cots at night. These individuals tend to function relatively well. Many are recently homeless and therefore likely to be less exhausted and worn than people at the other shelter sites.

Our team is present nineteen hours and sees about fifty people each week.

In providing on-site shelter care, we use a three-tier approach:

1. *Outreach*. Most of the time we allow people at the shelters to approach the team. Sometimes we aggressively seek out a particular person if it is medically warranted or if there is a medical emergency. Team members visit the dormitories to evaluate and assess general needs. At drop-in centers team members visit or make rounds at tables. Again, most assessment is done during casual interaction; many clients do not realize they are being assessed.

2. *Satellite or outreach clinic*. This is a specific area at a shelter, which should be large enough to accommodate several staff members. We attempt to maintain established hours of operation and stable assignment of personnel. Most teams consist of physicians, registered nurses, social workers. Some have case aides. The composition of each team varies according to the needs at individual shelters. There are two types of teams, the roving or traveling team and the stationary team.

All health stations have basic equipment: sink, examination table, and screening tools such as ophthalmoscope, otoscope, sphygmomanometer, stethoscope, and flashlights. Additional equipment may include electrocardiograph machines, blood-drawing instruments, charts (locked to insure confidentiality), and supplies such as bandages, gauzes, cleaning solutions, and gowns.

Communication among all agencies is essential. Thus a system is maintained to record daily activities—such as initial medical problem, treatment, and follow-up plans—and to communicate them to shelter staff and other involved agencies. Referral forms for interdepartment and interagency utilization are provided. And interagency meetings are scheduled on a regular basis.

3. *Traditional clinic or outpatient department.* This is for those people, SRO or shelter in origin, who are ready to learn to deal properly with the hospital system. The social worker and other members on the team advocate and act as liaison between outpatient staff, hospital administration, and clients. During this process outpatient staff are educated and are sensitized to the needs of the homeless. They have been quite helpful when the outreach staff is unavailable.

There are two primary care clinics at Saint Vincent's Hospital designed to meet the needs of clients in SRO hotels and shelters. A specific area is designated for the SRO/shelter clinic in proximity to the mainstream clinic. Based on our 1983 log book, there was an appointment compliance rate of 75.3 percent for all shelter and SRO patients. The average compliance rate for regular primary clinics is 70 percent. The success of these SRO clinics can be attributed to the following:

- The same health care staff that provide services at the outreach site are at the clinic session.
- The clients are familiar with and have developed a trusting relationship with outreach staff members and come to the clinic because of that relationship.
- Just as at the outreach sites, social workers act as case managers and are essential. They troubleshoot, help curb poor impulse control, and calm clients who are hostile or anxious.

Hospitalization

When a client is admitted to the hospital, the outreach team follows his/her course of treatment. There is an open channel of communication with house staff, inpatient social workers, and nurses. We can review the charts and add pertinent information. It is imperative that we visit clients; they welcome and appreciate a visit from a friendly, familiar face, someone they know and trust.

Convalescence

For many illnesses, time is needed after hospitalization for full recuperation. For many homeless people, this interim period is nonexistent. To return them to drop-in centers or shelters without beds seems inhumane but sometimes there is no alternative. The outreach staff tries to get patients discharged to a place with beds, and if it is a shelter that the team is not involved with, to connect them with another health team or have them return to the site or clinic for follow-up care.

Transportation

Many individuals do not keep appointments because they lack money to pay for transportation. Therefore, we provide transportation for those who have clinic appointments or scheduled diagnostic procedures.

If a vehicle is unavailable, or if the client is reliable, tokens are given so the client can take public transportation, with a promise that scheduled appointments will be kept. On occasion, we inform clients that a team member will meet them at the scheduled appointment.

PROBLEMS WITH CASE MANAGEMENT

There has been a great deal of discussion regarding the transient nature of this population. When they are absent from the shelter or SRO, medical care or psychosocial counseling is interrupted. Alcoholic binges, psychiatric episodes, and lost medications cause setbacks. The medical team is unable to complete health assessment, such as tuberculosis screening, when the client fails to show up two days after the skin test has been given. The time and energy invested by the various team members are substantial, but the challenge to bridge the gap in care, because it can be done, is a motivating factor that gives the staff energy to persevere.

REFERENCES

1. Killcommons, P. Paper presented at Saint Vincent's Hospital based on SRO program, 1974.
2. Brickner PW, Greenbaum D, Kaufman A, O'Donnell F, O'Brian JT, Scalice R, Scandizzo J, Sullivan T. A clinic for male derelicts. Ann Int Med. 1972; 77:565.
3. Brickner PW, Kaufman A. Heart disease in homeless men. Bull NY Acad Med. 1973; 49:475–84.
4. Leichter FS. Single room occupancy hotels: no rooms for rent, a plan for state action. Office of State Senator Leichter, New York, March 1980.
5. Jorgen R, Crowell R. SRO service program demographic study. New York: New York City Human Resources Administration, 1979.
6. Koop E, Murphy K. Lower-priced hotels. New York: New York City Human Resources Administration, 1978.
7. Baxter E, Hopper K: Private lives/public spaces. New York: New York Community Service Society, 1981.

23

Springfield, Massachusetts: The Sisters of Providence Health Care for the Homeless Program

Sister Julie Crane

Several months ago, while working as a server in a local soup kitchen, I became aware of a whole new population—people of no special age or background; people with no specific address, who spent their days and nights on the streets around town and who came to the soup kitchen at 5:00 P.M. for supper. Not everyone was poorly dressed, and the mixtures of colors and languages did not make any difference. They all had one thing in common: they were street people and they were hungry. I spent a lot of evenings there, just helping to serve supper, yet I could see the other needs in these people. The street people were glad to see each other for supper. When they left, I stood at the door to say good night and to wish them a safe night. For weeks I pondered these people.

Until that time, I really had not looked at the people who passed me on the street, but one day I noticed more and more soup-kitchen people around town. More and more shelters were opening. The governor was talking about the homeless. Their numbers were on the rise. I looked at these people and knew I had to do something about the needs they did not mention, but that I could easily see.

HEALTH CARE PROBLEMS OF
STREET PEOPLE

Their health and social needs were more difficult to assess than their numbers. They displayed a wide variety of nutritional problems, alcohol and substance abuse, infection and chronic disease. And so at the soup kitchen we started a simple medical clinic: we took blood pressures and gave foot soaks. Saying "how are you" and "good night" turned into looking at lacerations and counseling pregnant women, referring clients to detox and doing medication checks. This simple evening of caring slowly developed into the Sisters of Providence Health Care for the Homeless, formally established on July 5, 1983.

In the first six months 339 people had been cared for, with 1020 subsequent visits, resulting in a total of 1359 visits over the period extending through December 31, 1983. Tables 23.1–23.4, presented later in the article, display information on the services that have been provided to date. They bear testimony to the formerly unmet needs of the homeless.

Like other major urban areas, Springfield has a significant population of homeless people. Their living situation results from factors that range from alcohol abuse to mental illness, including recent state efforts at deinstitutionalization. According to the 1980 census, the population of Springfield is 152,319; however, since this population count is based on a residential survey, the number of homeless or "street people" is difficult to estimate. Several social service providers indicate that there are at least 500 homeless residents in Springfield who utilize various food, shelter, and SRO (single-room-occupancy) services.

Neither the 1979 State Health Plan nor the 1983 Draft State Health Plan addresses the health care needs of the homeless population. Rather, the plans recommend future health care services or discuss public policy issues that at best would have indirect impact on the target population. However, awareness of the needs of the homeless is increasing. In his January 1983 inaugural address, Massachusetts Governor Michael Dukakis named assistance to the homeless people in our state as a top priority of his administration.

Health care problems plague the homeless. These include poor hygiene, lack of dental care, weight problems, severe smoking habits, and dermatological disorders. Deinstitutionalization has dramatically increased the presence on the street of people with uncontrolled psychiatric problems, and today this population is more obvious than ever. Shelters are crowded with people who once lived in institutions, where their activities could be monitored and medications administered with consistency. More and more of these people are living on the streets and not being looked after; consequently, they present a significant problem to the shelters where they seek refuge. The lack of kitchen facilities is often related to their nutritional deficiencies. Weight problems are prevalent: it is cheaper and easier to have a cup of hot chocolate and a few donuts than it is to make a substantial meal. Getting food on an erratic basis, from wherever one can, also contributes to health problems. Boredom and lack of structured activities have led this population to be particularly heavy smokers. Many of the people have productive coughs and difficulties with breathing. Dermatological problems stem from inaccessibility to laundry products and facilities.

Diabetes mellitus is a difficult health care problem for the street person, and a surprising number of our clients are diabetic. Most of them are maintained on insulin. A diabetic diet is unheard of. The first concern of the homeless is getting something to eat rather than the ratio of fats to carbohydrates in their diets. Skin breakdown and ulceration compound the diabetic's problem, especially when there are no bathing facilities.

Many of our clients have a history of seizures and are on anticonvulsant drug therapy. Those who have had seizures since early childhood attribute them to elevated fever during a bout with measles, while those with adult onset attribute them to alcoholism and traumatic injury to the head. Compliance with Dilantin®, phenobarbital, or Tegretol® regimens is unpredictable and is complicated by alcohol consumption.

The changing seasons bring new health problems. As summer brings poison ivy, winter brings frostbite. For the street person, winter in the East is a long and dreaded time of the year. Large crates are prized possessions; these and heat coming up from street grates are sometimes the only sources of warmth. It is common to read in the newspapers of a street person being found dead behind the local school or church, a person no one had ever seen before.

Upper respiratory infections are always more frequent in the winter. Temperature checks, lung sounds, and simple preparations of Tylenol© and cough medicine are, for the most part, the remedies that we provide, along with warm clothing and a place out of the cold, always welcome relief until spring comes again.

Street life is violent. The wounds and lacerations that result expose excellent media for infections. Soap and water scrubs and clean dressings with an antibiotic ointment keep the injured area protected, but the cause of violence is often related to alcoholism.

The incidence of alcoholism is alarming among the street people.

This city houses a large population at the detox center, and it is always full. The detox success rate for this population is not good. The same people I have taken to detox return to the soup kitchen asking again: "Sister, will you take me to detox?"

Schizophrenic and manic-depressive clients are present in great numbers, and follow-up care is lacking. My experience is that they are either out of or feel that they no longer need medication and do not want to have any psychiatric follow-up. They abandon their usual address and become street wanderers. Their social workers do not know where they are. The schizophrenic client who is also a hard core drug user presents even greater problems, because of the reaction produced by the combination of psychotropic and street drugs.

Hypertension is always a big problem with the street person. As with the diabetic, diet is not considered important and medication is taken variably.

We are frequently aware of the location of clients who are known to have had tuberculosis and are not presenting themselves for routine examinations, treatment, or follow-up. We notify the health department of the whereabouts of these clients or bring them to the TB clinic ourselves. We look for them regularly and attempt to make sure they follow treatment.

The list of problems is extensive for this population and would be incomplete without mention of the physical and emotional exhaustion they experience. Lack of a home, lack of finances or support, all greatly decrease people's defenses, and they become much more vulnerable to a myriad of health problems.

The need for early medical intervention for these people is obvious. Otherwise their medical problems become more severe, and eventually hospitalization is necessary. Increased inconvenience and/or discomfort for the patient, as well as the use of increasingly expensive health care resources, result. Preventive health care initiatives like Health Care for the Homeless can be very successful in avoiding the need for inpatient care.

The goal of Sisters of Providence Health Care for the Homeless is to improve the health status of the homeless of Springfield through preventive care. Each of the family shelters, the men's shelter, and the women's shelter are visited daily. Late afternoon visits to the soup kitchen and throughout the day to local hangout spots provide health care opportunities for those who do not live at the shelters. Those problems that the nurse practitioner cannot handle are referred to volunteer doctors and dentists. Close contact with other referral agencies encourages appointments and essential follow-up.

During its first six months of operation, Health Care for the Homeless utilized several program sites and referral agencies.

Jefferson Street, operated by the Open Pantry, a food distribution organization, provides a home for women and children, whereas Cummings Memorial is for men only. Prospect Street and the Springfield Rescue Mission look after the housing needs of men, women, and children. The unit run by the Salvation Army, although not regarded as a shelter, provides a residence as well as a rehabilitation center for recovering alcoholics. Loaves and Fishes insures a nightly meal, and the Women's Place provides care for women and children who would otherwise have no place to stay during the day.

Although many of the needs of street people are medically related, there are multiple other agencies or referrals needed by this population. (See Tables 23.1 and 23.2.)

Table 23.3 displays the number of visits made and describes the client population served by Health Care for the Homeless during its first six months of operation. Part A shows the total number of visits by site and Part B the number of clients by population subgroups and the average number of visits per client. Loaves and Fishes incorporates the Women's Place in the utilization statistics. The Salvation Army statistics reflect only the month of December 1983, as their services were not provided until then.

Table 23.4 lists the diagnoses and number of incidences identified during the first six months of operation.

All cases referred to another health care provider or social service agency are displayed in Table 23.2, Section A. The clinical reasons for inpatient hospitalization are listed in Section B.

PROGRAM STAFFING AND OPERATION

The program director is a family nurse practitioner, licensed in Massachusetts, and the main provider of services since the program's inception. She is responsible for the overall direction of the program, and sees clients/patients daily for routine physical exams, assessments, and plans. She supervises staff, student interns, and volunteers and coordinates a schedule of site visits to the various locations.

The director represents Health Care for the Homeless throughout the community and accepts speaking engagements whenever possible.

She manages the program budget and is responsible for identifying appropriate funding sources. She also assesses the feasibility of providing health services to the homeless in other municipalities.

Table 23.1. Program Sites and Referral Agencies, July–December 1983 (Sisters of Providence Health Care for the Homeless)

Program Sites
  Jefferson Street Shelter
  Prospect Street Shelter
  Springfield Rescue Mission
  Cummings Memorial
  Salvation Army
  Loaves and Fishes
  Women's Place

Referral Agencies
  Open Pantry
  Mercy Hospital Social Services
  Mercy Emergency Room
  Police Department
  Health Department
  VNA
  Social Services (Bay Street)
  Wesson Memorial Medical & Surgical Clinics,
    ER and VD Clinic
  Housing Allowance Program
  Springfield Developmental Center
  Service Coordination Program
  Veteran's Administration
  Springfield Welfare
  Food Stamp Office
  Social Security
  Community Care
  Vocational Rehabilitation
  Council of Churches
  Baystate Pediatric Unit
  Detoxification Center

The director is assisted by a staff of registered nurses, who are currently scheduled to rotate through the program based on the hours they are willing to volunteer. They receive assignments of shelters and sites to be visited at the start of each day. At present, volunteer nurses provide basic health assessment, treatment, and education. Nurses also perform all related duties that contribute to assessing and alleviating the clients' medical conditions.

Table 23.2. **Referrals to Other Agencies, July–December 1983 (Sisters of Providence Health Care for the Homeless)**

A. Type of Referral Agency	Number of Referrals
Hospital Emergency Room	15
Hospital Clinic	9
Private Physician (Total)	10
Specialists: Dermatology	3
Ophthalmology	1
Internal Medicine	1
Orthopedics	2
Surgery	1
Dentist	1
Nursing Home	5
Mental Health Center	10
Lawyer	1
City Hall	1
Detox	4
Massachusetts Department of Rehabilitation	1
Social Security	2
Division of Social Service	1
Massachusetts Association for the Blind	1
Lions Club	1
School	1
Loaves and Fishes	1
Open Pantry	4
Welfare	1
Shelter	1
Probate Court	1
Court Cases	1
Law Enforcement	1
Child and Family Services	3
Total	84

B. Inpatient Hospitalizations

1. Diabetes—Diarrhea	7. Carcinoma of the Testicle
2. Psychiatric Disorder	8. Congestive Heart Failure
3. Colostomy	9. Diabetes
4. Kidney Stones	10. Colostomy Closure
5. Hypertension	11. Hepatitis
6. Abdominal Pain	12. Diabetes
	13. Diabetes

Table 23.3.   Utilization Statistics, July–December 1983 (Sisters of Providence Health Care for the Homeless)

A. Sites						
	Loaves and Fishes	*Taylor Street*	*Prospect Street*	*Jeff Street*	*Bliss Street and Other*	*Salvation Army*	*Total*
Total number visits	520	321	180	104	209	25	1,359

B. Client Population

Client Population Served

Adult Males	233
Adult Females	78
Children	28
Total	339

Average Number of Visits Per Client

Adult Males	233/936 = 4.0 Visits/Male
Adult Females	78/311 = 4.0 Visits/Female
Children	28/112 = 4.0 Visits/Child
Total	339/1,359 = 4.0 Visits/Client

Appointments for follow-up visits to physicians, dentists, or nurse practitioners are noted. Transportation is provided, and the client is accompanied to the appointment whenever possible. Follow-up care information is always obtained and followed precisely. We coordinate efforts with other local agencies, such as the Visiting Nurses and Welfare Office, so that the clients will be in touch with agencies that will benefit them to the full.

Nurses visit clients who are recuperating at the hospital and prepare for their disposition upon discharge with the social service department.

The nurses are assisted by student nurses, for whom a rotation schedule has been initiated. This program offers an opportunity for students to gain a new perspective on the provision of health care while giving additional support to the paid staff. A similar internship program for social work students is planned for the coming year.

There is one secretary who collects statistics. Medical consultation, dental care, and podiatry services are provided by volunteers.

Table 23.4. Major Diagnoses Identified, July–December 1983 (Sisters of Providence Health Care for the Homeless)

Diagnoses	Number of Incidences
Hypertension	211
Foot and leg care and disorders	189
Physical examinations	149
Psychiatric problems	94
Referrals	84
Dermatological problems	63
Dressing changes	60
Lacerations	54
Flu and cold symptoms	52
Alcoholism	48
Eye, ear, nose, and throat problems	46
Diabetes Mellitus	36
Cardiac problems	35
GI problems	29
Abdominal problems	23
Muscle strains	23
Skin tests and reading	20
Colostomies	19
Drug problems	15
Kidney problems	12
Pregnancies	9
Fractures	11
Pediculosis	8
Toothaches	8
Epilepsy	12
Fevers of undetermined origin	5
Puncture wounds	5
Burns	4
Lymphadenopathy	4
Vaginitis	4
Breast tumors	3
Ecchymosis	3
Edema	3
Venereal diseases	3
Headaches	2
Physical abuse	2
Testicular carcinoma	2
Arthritis	1
Asthma	1
Cellulitis	1
Infection, severe	1
Immunization	1
Pseudocyesis	1
Syncope	1
Tuberculosis	1
Urethral discharge	1
Total	1,359

Health Care for the Homeless currently operates ten hours a day, five days a week. Weekend coverage is under consideration, depending upon the identified needs in the Springfield area. At present this program is operated only in Springfield; it is anticipated that experience will direct us to other areas of need in the future.

Two paid, twenty-hour-per-week nursing positions are proposed for September 1984 to alleviate the increasing demand for clinical services. Volunteers have played a major role in this program to date, and it is hoped they will continue to do so; yet there is now a need for more consistent nurse availability.

More sites are requesting health services as word of their availability spreads amongst the street people. Greater opportunity for one-to-one contact with patients, more time to investigate individual clients' problems, stronger liaison with community referral agencies, and increased dependability of paid staff will result from the proposed nursing positions.

Response to the clients' identified diseases is a major concern in the operation of this kind of program. By offering health screening, assessment, treatment, and education service, the provider is responsible for referring the patient/client to an appropriate source of care. The target population generally needs prompt care, but not emergency services. If program personnel feel emergency services are required, clients are transferred to the local emergency room of their choice. Patients admitted to the hospital are seen by representatives of the Social Service Department for eligibility assessment and follow-up. Those with disorders that do not require acute hospitalization are scheduled for a follow-up visit at the site where they were identified, or at another site in the program. Flexibility must be maintained so that the most appropriate health care service can be provided for the patient in need.

SUMMARY

The Sisters of Providence currently sponsor health care programs for the homeless and destitute in Springfield, Massachusetts. Services include health assessment, health education, treatment, nutritional counseling, alcohol counseling, and referral for emergency health services. The experience of the initial six months of operation indicates that there are several hundred homeless persons who are in need and can be served each year. Services are currently provided at the transients' congregating sites by a nurse practitioner, volunteer nurses, and physicians.

The health care problems of the street people will persist, and so will the preventive care we have initiated. We cannot measure our success by statistics; rather, success is measured by the pain and illness that we are able to prevent.

As admirable as these goals may be, when we are faced with their enormity and complexity, we wonder if we can ever achieve them. We begin each day where we are, by doing what we can individually, and by joining with others with related concerns to work for solutions that maximize available resources for those in great need.

24

Washington, D.C.: The Zacchaeus Clinic— A Model of Health Care for Homeless Persons

Eve Bargmann

Zaccheus Clinic is a free medical clinic in inner-city Washington, D.C. It was opened in February 1974 in response to the unmet health needs of homeless persons coming to the local soup kitchen. Getting the clinic on its feet required the joint efforts of several churches, a group (the Community for Creative Nonviolence) committed to providing help for the homeless, and local physicians and other health professionals.

The clinic is funded entirely by donations from individuals, churches, and community groups, supplemented by small grants. It receives no federal or local government money. The current budget is approximately $70,000 per year, which pays for staff salaries, medications, laboratory work, malpractice insurance, office and laboratory supplies, and all operating expenses.

Four full-time paid staff work at the clinic: a physician, two administrative coordinators, and a social worker/outreach worker. In addition, approximately 100 people work at the clinic as volunteers. Walk-in clinics on Tuesday and Thursday evenings and Saturday mornings are staffed largely by volunteers, who work as receptionists at the front desk, do laboratory tests and blood drawing, take patients' histories and vital signs, and dispense prescribed medications. At least one of the twelve volunteer physicians works at each clinic session; as a rule, a physician sees each patient. Other volunteers include nurses, nurse practitioners, physicians' assistants, interested community members, and patients; each is oriented at the clinic and given further training on the job and at special sessions.

In addition to services at walk-in clinics, medical care is offered in the daytime by appointment. Here, a clinic physician sees patients who need physical examinations, more extensive evaluation, or ongoing care for long-term problems.

To fill the need for consultants, clinic volunteers wrote to subspecialists in the District, asking them to see up to one clinic patient each month free of charge. Around sixty have agreed to do so and have seen and treated the clinic's patients as needed for many years. These include ophthalmologists, otolaryngologists, orthopedists, gynecologists, podiatrists, dentists, neurologists, gastroenterologists, general surgeons, a cardiologist, and an optometrist.

The clinic does some laboratory work on-site. A local laboratory has donated its services and does not charge for several of the tests that the clinic would otherwise need to send out and pay for. The city laboratory donates culture plates as well as pap smears and blood tests for syphilis.

MEDICAL CARE FOR HOMELESS PEOPLE IN WASHINGTON, D.C.

Five small community clinics in the District offer health care to poor persons, including the homeless. Zacchaeus Clinic is one of these. It offers care and medications at no charge. The four other clinics charge on a sliding scale; one of them carries a limited stock of medications. Other available resources are the District's public health clinics, which also charge on a sliding scale; hospital emergency rooms; D.C. General Hospital, a public hospital; and Saint Elizabeth's Hospital, a federally funded mental institution.

The Community for Creative Nonviolence has opened a twelve-bed infirmary for homeless persons with acute medical problems. Because almost all shelters require their guests to spend the day outside, places like this infirmary are essential to offer twenty-four hour shelter, running water, and food to homeless persons weakened by illness.

More often than not, only those who actively seek medical care receive it. These people tend to go to a hospital emergency room or to one of the community clinics. Most find the public health clinics and hospital-based clinics too forbidding.

DEMOGRAPHICS OF CLINIC PATIENTS

Zacchaeus Clinic sees not only homeless people, but also other indigent people. Nevertheless, the clinic is a major source of care for the homeless, who generally view it as open and accessible. It is free and close to a number of shelters and drop-in centers. The clinic shares a block with three women's shelters, a family shelter, a distributor of free food and clothing, and a women's day center. It is two blocks from the Central Union Mission and three blocks from another women's day center.

Zacchaeus Clinic sees approximately 4000 patients per year. Each year, the clinic sees between 700 and 1300 new patients; since 1974, it has served approximately 9000 individuals.

The clinic's patients are 76 percent black, 20 percent white, and 4 percent other races and nationalities. A survey done in 1980 found the median family income of clinic patients to be $300 per month. Most do not have Medicare, Medicaid, or other health insurance.

Approximately 15 percent of patients at Zacchaeus Clinic are homeless. Slightly more than half of these (54 percent) are women. The unusually large proportion of women probably reflects the fact that three women's shelters and a women's day center are located on the same block as the clinic.

Homeless patients at the clinic range in age from eighteen (the clinic sees only adults) to over sixty. The median age of homeless patients is thirty-nine.

The major health problems of a sample of the clinic's homeless patients are listed in Table 24.1. Most patients have multiple health problems.

As the table shows, homeless patients presented with a full range of medical problems. Many did suffer from "illnesses of the destitute,"[1] such as lice, tuberculosis, alcoholism, and psychological problems, but many more presented with such common medical problems as respiratory infections, made more common by exposure and malnutrition. The striking prevalence of anemia probably reflects malnutrition as well as chronic illness.

THE CLINIC'S THREE GOALS

A discussion of the clinic can best be organized around its three officially adopted goals. These are:

- to provide quality health care with dignity to persons in the area;

Table 24.1. Major Health Problems of Homeless Patients

Medical Condition	Prevalence
Alcohol abuse (current or past)*	40%
Respiratory infections	30%
Anemia	22%
Hypertension	20%
Major mental illness	18%
Injuries	18%
Gynecologic problems	16%
Obesity	12%
Miscellaneous dermatologic problems	12%

Problems seen in 5 to 10 percent of patients:

Urinary	Acute dental	Foot problems
Gastrointestinal	Seizures	Pregnancy
Lice/Scabies	Gonorrhea	Soft tissue infection
Musculoskeletal pain (not injury)		

Problems seen in fewer than 5 percent of patients:

Tuberculosis	Illegal drug use	General examination
Glaucoma	Arthritis	Heart disease
Duodenal ulcer	Chronic obstructive	Headache
Phlebitis	pulmonary disease	Hand contracture
Pancreatitis	Weight loss	Hypercholesterolemia
Hand numbness	Leg edema	

*This figure includes binge drinkers and others who may not be drinking at the time of their visit to the clinic. Approximately three-quarters of this sample had an active alcohol problem at the time they were seen.

- to involve patients and providers equally in decisions, both individually and in the clinic as a whole; and
- to help one another change systems that impede quality health care from being given with dignity.

Quality and Dignity

Some of the clinic's efforts to provide quality health care have already been described. The work of two staff coordinators helps achieve the quality care goal. Coordinators are present at each clinic session. In addition to administrative duties, they review each patient's chart the day after he or she is seen. They make sure that all problems have been dealt with; record and review all laboratory test results and call patients back if their laboratory tests were abnormal; make appointments for patients with consultants and help the patients get to these appointments; and contact patients who did not come for scheduled return visits. Intensive follow-up is an essential part of ongoing care at the clinic.

Equally important in effecting quality care at the clinic is a full-time staff social worker/outreach worker. This person helps patients procure any government assistance to which they are entitled, such as Medicaid and food stamps; helps patients find housing, emergency shelter, or jobs; counsels those with various crises or drug or alcohol problems and refers them to other agencies when needed; coordinates the pre-natal clinic, which includes homeless women among its patients; and maintains contact with other community agencies and policy-making groups.

Providing quality—or even adequate—medical care to these in-digent patients also requires that they receive all needed medications free of charge. For those without money or Medicaid, a prescription is no more than a piece of paper. A steady stream of patients comes to the clinic because they cannot afford medications for such long-term problems as hypertension, diabetes mellitus, and cardiac disease; they want to take care of their health, but find medications simply out of the range of their budgets.

An integral part of each volunteer's orientation is an emphatic intro-duction to the clinic policy of treating patients with dignity and respect, as equals and persons of worth. The peer pressure of other volunteers further encourages this behavior.

Because homeless people in particular are suspicious of bureaucracy and regulations, the clinic keeps rules to a minimum. No patient is asked to fill out forms, answer questions about his or her income or assets, or present an ID. The only rules are:

- Patients will not be seen while they are intoxicated.
- They may not drink or take street drugs while in the clinic.
- They are expected to treat each other with respect, as those at the clinic treat them. This means, at a minimum, that they should not be verbally or physically abusive.

Patient Involvement

The clinic's second goal is to involve patients and providers equally in decisions, both individually and in the clinic as a whole.

Patient involvement in individual decisions means that patients are

expected to share in decisions about their health and to take responsibility for those decisions and for their health. Clinic staff and volunteers continuously work to educate patients and help them make healthier choices in their lives; patients are expected to work at this as well.

Patients are involved in clinic decisions and activities in many ways.
Patients serve on the clinic's steering committee. With active encouragement from the clinic staff (including offering free food, announcing
meetings at walk-in clinics, and calling individual patients), patients
come to general clinic meetings, where all major clinic decisions are
made. Patients also serve as volunteers at the clinic; they work in the
laboratory, at the front desk, in the pharmacy, and see other patients
as patient advocates.

Involving patients is important to the well-being of both patients
and the clinic. Recently, someone put a brick through the clinic's front
window. Because installment of another window would have been pro-
hibitively expensive, the staff chose to install the window itself. As one
of the coordinators attempted to do so, a homeless man from the
Gospel Mission came by and offered advice. After a while, he took off
his coat—actually, several coats—and began to put in the window himself. He had worked for twenty years as a glazier, putting windows into
public schools, and he did a lovely job with whatever cast-off materials
he could find in the clinic basement. When he finished, he seemed to
stand a foot taller—and some of the clinic's workers left with a totally
new view of homeless people.

Patients at the clinic need to see themselves as equal participants
with something to offer, not as recipients of charity. The clinic in turn
depends on patients for their help and for their understanding of the
community and its needs; it depends on them to teach other volunteers
and to keep the clinic on course.

Working to Change Systems

The clinic's third goal is to work to change systems that keep people
from receiving quality health care and from being treated with dignity.
This goal mandates that the clinic not simply offer whatever health care
it can to the homeless and stop there. The clinic must deal with the
larger problems that cause and perpetuate homelessness and poverty.

John was forty-five years old, lived on the city's heat grates, and
drank heavily. He had diabetes mellitus, hypertension, large bunions,
and small shoes. The ulcer on one of his feet exposed the bone.

Step one for John—not an easy one—was to persuade him to stop drinking. One way of encouraging this was to open the clinic to him on a daily basis to allow him to clean, soak, and dress his feet, supplemented by debriding by the clinic physician. This stopped the ulcer from enlarging; but he was still on his feet and in his shoes much of the day, and the ulcer did not improve.

Step two was to find him twenty-four-hour shelter and a better pair of shoes. The Community for Creative Nonviolence, which runs a hospitality house for people who are homeless and ill, provided both. While he stayed there, his ulcer improved dramatically. But when he again moved out for a time, all improvement stopped. His ulcer did not heal until almost three months later—shortly after he had found another twenty-four-hour lodging place.

John now lives in an apartment and works at a hotel. He still comes to the clinic regularly for treatment of his high blood pressure and diabetes.

The message from John, and from many others like him, is that health workers cannot deal with the medical needs of individual homeless people without first finding them safe, warm lodging and nutritious food. This means working closely with shelters, soup kitchens, and other community resources and, in the long run, helping these patients find permanent lodging and a steady source of food; helping them find work if they can work or get disability or public assistance if they cannot.

This is even more the case for women, as homelessness is rapidly becoming an equal opportunity problem.[2] Homeless women are intensely vulnerable. Most have been robbed, many have been assaulted, and a substantial number have been raped. Many have untreated psychological problems. Until they are out of danger, treating their lice and burns—not to mention their high blood pressure—is an exercise in futility.

Helping homeless people as a group means working in the community to increase their access to resources of all kinds, and working to deal with the larger problems of scarce resources. One clinic—or two or ten—cannot begin to meet the needs of Washington's homeless. Washington, like other cities, still has an incredible shortage of shelter beds, far too few low-income housing units, almost no secondary housing, little mental health care for poor persons, and even less dental care. The only hospital that offers inpatient psychiatric care for persons who cannot pay is eliminating ever more beds, adding to the already overwhelming problem of deinstitutionalization. The city has far fewer jobs than it has people, and poverty is widespread. Physical and mental health care and social services outreach to homeless people are still infinitesimal compared to the need. The city government can do far more than it is doing to provide health care to homeless people. The city government provides care through D.C. General Hospital, the only hospital consistently open to those unable to pay. But those who do not want to be hospitalized—and many homeless people do not seek hospitalization until they are desperately ill—tend to avoid the city-run outreach clinics as well. A survey of groups dealing with homeless people—shelters, soup kitchens, and day centers—found that these people most often go for medical care to hospital emergency rooms or to one of the small community clinics, including Zacchaeus Clinic.

Long waits, paperwork and other requirements, being shuffled from place to place, and impersonal treatment are not well tolerated by homeless people. Such barriers are common in city clinics, and they often arise naturally—from the need for documentation, from under-staffing, from inadequate funds, from low staff morale. But these barriers must be overcome or circumvented to make city clinics accessible to homeless people.

Ideally, a specific person at each clinic could be assigned to serve as a contact person for homeless patients. This person:

- would have no duties that have a higher priority than helping homeless patients, so that other tasks would not prevent him or her from taking the time needed with these people;
- would help homeless patients negotiate the clinic's system as quickly and as smoothly as possible;
- would help homeless persons secure shelter, food, and social services;
- would maintain contact with agencies serving homeless persons, establishing a working link between these agencies and the clinic; and
- would arrange for outreach to homeless persons in need of health care.

Some concerned and well-intentioned city employees have developed a habit of impotence over the years, a conviction that government systems are so difficult to change that the struggle is not even worth the attempt. Assigning the role of contact person for the homeless to one of these people, or to someone already burdened with other duties, will not accomplish the task. Each contact person must not only be able to make the existing health care system work better, but must be dedicated to that end. Others working at the clinics also need to become convinced that change is possible. This arrangement could ultimately provide a model for improving the access of all indigent people—not only those who are homeless—to health care and social services.

DIRECTIONS FOR CHANGE

All those who work with homeless people, and all those genuinely concerned about the plight of the homeless, must speak out for long-term solutions. We must work to:

- increase the range of services available to homeless and other indigent people, and improve the access of indigent people to these services;
- increase the housing available to indigent persons—shelters, secondary housing, and low-income housing;
- make systems such as Supplemental Security Income and Medicaid more accessible to those who are entitled to help, but often do not get it;
- ensure that mentally ill persons receive both ongoing mental health care and housing appropriate for them; and
- mitigate the larger problems—unemployment, lack of job training, lack of education, lack of hope—which cause and perpetuate poverty and homelessness in our country.

As Zacchaeus Clinic shows, much can be done with little money and a few dedicated and enthusiastic people. Far more can, and must, be done. Washington, D.C., has over 1000 psychiatrists[3]—more psychiatrists per capita than any other city in the country—and almost no mental health services for homeless people. Even shelters with psychiatric emergencies often have nowhere to turn. If only a fraction of Washington's psychiatrists could be recruited to give a small amount of time, the city would increase the availability of these desperately needed services without unduly burdening any one person.

Dental care could also be expanded by opening a dental clinic staffed by volunteer dentists. Several dentists have called the clinic looking for places where they can volunteer, and there are probably others willing to do so as well.

Health care workers and social workers should also go regularly to shelters, soup kitchens, and heating grates to offer health screening, referral, first aid, and social services. Volunteers, coordinated by one or a few paid staff, could also provide such services.

The Zacchaeus Clinic may be a model, but it is one small clinic. It must be part of a much larger effort. Volunteers working alone cannot do all that needs to be done. We must make sure that our services extend, that our efforts engender other efforts, that people will have access not only to whatever few services we can provide, not only to limited health care if they know where to find it, but also to the rights and services and dignity to which they all are entitled. That is our hope and our goal.

REFERENCES

1. Hewetson J. Homeless people as an at-risk group. Proc Roy Soc Med. 1975; 68:9–13.
2. Slavinsky AT, Cousins A. Homeless women. Nursing Outlook. 1982; 30: 358–62.
3. Torrey EF. The real twilight zone. Washington Post. August 26, 1983.

Index ————————————————————